THE PALLIATIVE CARE CHRONICLES

MEET PEARL, DALE, AND DR. LEA

DR. GERALD HARRIMAN

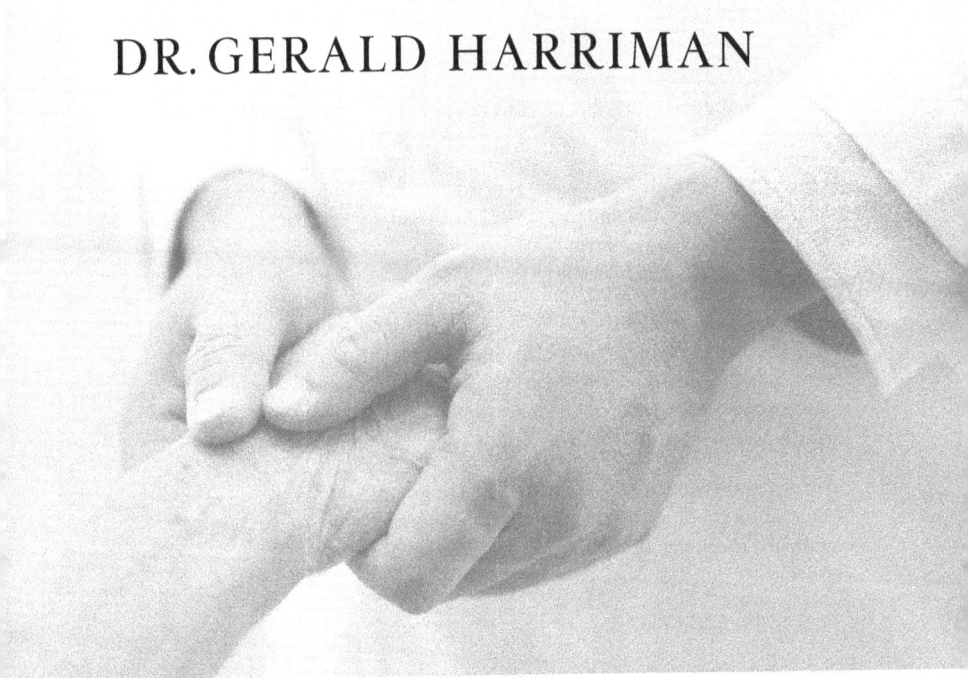

credo
house publishers

Published in the United States of America by Credo House Publishers,
a division of Credo Communications LLC, Grand Rapids, Michigan
credohousepublishers.com

Although Dr. Gerald A. Harriman is a physician, he is not your
physician. The content of this book is not intended to be a substitute
for professional medical advice, diagnosis, or treatment. Always
consult with a qualified healthcare professional for any questions you
may have regarding a specific medical condition or before making
any decisions related to your health or treatment.

The medical scenarios, characters, and treatments depicted do not
represent a specific patient, though they may be based on the actual
medical experience of the author. Any resemblance to real people
or events is coincidental.

ISBN: 978-1-62586-347-8

Cover and interior design by Sharon VanLoozenoord
Editing by Donna Huisjen

Printed in the United States of America

First Edition

CONTENTS

PREFACE

THIS book is written in the form of a story, featuring many conversations between the patient and the doctor who is providing comfort care. I wrote it this way as creative nonfiction to inform the reader in the context of patient stories about how palliative care visits unfold and what is included in them. The medical information is accurate as of the time the book was written, while the patient information actually combines details from several people, helping to secure patient privacy while providing a wider view by focusing on two composite patients who together encapsulate the experiences of a handful. Each chapter is named after one of the two patients, the main topic of their visit, or a relevant topic if the material is not focused on a patient encounter.

Additionally, to assist with clarity the time interval since the last chapter for that patient is included to help the reader keep track of their story through the book. Interspersed among the patient care chapters are factual summary chapters on palliative care that pause the story to provide important information and help the reader better understand this kind of care. These will describe and expand on important aspects of palliative care that don't necessarily apply to the patient's specific story or conversation.

Palliative care mainly happens through conversation. In fact, it has been said that the most important medical instrument for palliative care is the chair. This means that the palliative care provider sits in a chair and has a conversation on an equal eye level with the patient, so that the doctor is not above or apart from the patient. Resorting to more formal terminology, this is less paternalistic and more autonomous for the patient.

The physician is in the same space as the patient to enhance the encounter experience for both and to encourage open back and forth dialogue. You could say that the conversation itself is the medical procedure, or the main part, of a palliative care patient visit. It is the "medical instrument" for the clinician to gain patient input and explain necessary medical information, as well as for the patient to share their symptoms and their response to treatment or therapies or to communicate their goals and feelings. In a real sense palliative care is about the physician exploring the patient's thoughts, emotions, wishes, and understanding during the visit.

A well-known medical proverb is that patients want not only to know and understand but to be known and understood. The quote is usually credited to Ralph G. Nichols, PhD, who has been called "the father of listening" (1916–2006). An American expert in communication, he has worked in education and psychology and has written *Are You Listening? The science of improving your listening ability for a better understanding of people* (1957).[1] Listening is an essential skill for effective communication that meets the patient's needs.

This book is not intended to review the concepts of understanding, patient autonomy, learning information, and judging decision making. If you want to read a good article that explains these ideas in a way that connects to medical decisions, I recommend a recent piece by Caitríona B. Cox, MB, titled *Patient Understanding: how should it be defined and assessed in clinical practice?*[2]

The conversation with the patient during the encounter is in some sense like a CT scan or MRI in that it provides a snapshot that allows the palliative care physician to visualize what's going on medically inside the patient. But it goes further in providing not only a structural picture but also a functional one. The discussion helps the palliative care physician see how the person is feeling and functioning.

A medical imaging test such as a CT scan or MRI shows the structure of body organs, tissues, or abnormal occurrences at a specific moment at the time of the scan, but it doesn't do a good job of revealing how well the organ is working. That's where dialogue comes in: the conversation with the patient is like a laboratory test to see how the body's inner workings are functioning. This works in much the same way as do measurements like BUN and creatinine for kidney function; hemoglobin (the amount of blood in the body) to help determine the degree of anemia; the oxygen saturation level to indicate the function and capacity of the lungs to exchange oxygen for carbon dioxide gases; or a tumor marker level to indicate the status of cancer recurrence.

When teaching doctors in training in this field, I would talk to them after a patient encounter, and we would break down the implications of the conversation. I might lead the discussion with prompts like, "Why did I ask that question? Did I pause and give the patient time to answer, rather than filling in the void of silence? How well did I explain complicated medical conditions or consequences so the patient could understand and make appropriate decisions?"

This would be the equivalent of a teaching surgeon talking about incisions, suturing, or techniques to operate on patients (e.g., "Why was the incision made this way? How do you close the incision in proper layers? How do you control bleeding during an operation? Or Why use this piece of equipment or a specific model for a knee replacement?"

It is important for doctors in palliative care to do this well, as this will be the difference between establishing trust or failing to do so, getting an answer or not, or being able to stay in the patient room or be thrown with an outburst like "How dare you talk to me about this topic?"

On a side note, in light of the serious talks we must have with patients, we will undoubtedly encounter situations in which patients or family members do not want to talk about these matters any longer, possibly after others have tried unsuccessfully to address them. That's why they've called in palliative care providers: to get the decision the medical team wants (e.g., to get the DNR order or prevent the feeding tube the family wants to have inserted in the patient or to get them to talk about a topic pertinent to their condition and case).

Unfortunately, there will be instances in which we are asked to leave the room—sometimes right away but at other times after we begin talking. But we doctors can take heart in the knowledge that this outcome actually means we're doing our job properly. We've made an effort to have the tough conversation. If it didn't go well this time, there might be other chances to try again—such as the next time the patient is hospitalized, if that happens. Timing is out of our control as families deal with the inevitable.

I also wanted to demonstrate how each patient is dealing internally with the conversations recorded between physician and patient (and family) in the story chapters. I use italics to indicate the patient's thought process. The identity of the speaker will be clear enough, so I will use the italics only to designate the speaker's (patient's or physician's or family member's) inner voice. More than one point of view may be presented in a chapter, but not in the same paragraph.

I wrote the book in this way because people enjoy reading or listening to stories. The goal is to present the principles of palliative care in an engaging manner, and you, the reader, can decide if the approach succeeds.

I list resources in the order in which they appear in the stories, as well as in the listing of sources in the back. At the time of writing the medical entries were considered to be relevant and up to date.

As a physician who specializes in hospice, palliative medicine, and family medicine, I want to clarify that the encounters described are fictional and do not intentionally represent any one specific person, although many of the situations and scenarios are based on real life events. Some creativity is used to add detail to the story and make the actual patients unrecognizable.

Any medical advice provided in the context of the story should not be used as a medical reference by the reader. It is important for the reader to talk to their own doctors about any medical questions, diagnosis, treatment, and information on health issues specific to their condition. Don't use this book as a resource to diagnose or treat medical issues.

I was inspired by two books for the writing style used in this one. The first is *Tuesdays with Morrie* by Mitch Albom. This nonfiction book tells the story of weekly talks between a former student (the author) and his respected professor, who was dying from a terminal illness. I enjoyed the format for conveying the story line and capturing the conversations and the depth of the emotions. The second is a well-known novel by John Steinbeck titled *The Grapes of Wrath*. Steinbeck made extensive use of the technique of interspersing narrative chapters (the story) with chapters providing important historical background information.

With that said, let's get started . . .

Dr. Gerald Harriman

PEARL and DR. LEA

INTRODUCTIONS

"GOOD morning. I'm Dr. Lea Glendale, and I go by Dr. Lea." She pronounced the name in a somewhat exaggerated manner, as it is properly pronounced: "Lay-Ah." "Nice to meet you. Pearl Murphy—is that correct?"

"Yes, Doctor, that's correct. You may call me Pearl—that's what I prefer."

"Thank you. I will. Your name is familiar to me. Have we met before?"

"Yes, in the hospital the last time I was there. I was quite sick. You took care of me as a consultant on their palliative care team. It was a few months back."

"Yes, yes, I remember now. We discovered we're both Irish, though only you are from the homeland, and that we both love custard pie and Notre Dame Irish football. I'm going to set down my tablet, shake your hand if that's okay, and then sit down. Please forgive me for not remembering you right off. I was finishing up my palliative care fellowship at that time. I've now graduated and joined the hospital's group, though I'm starting out in clinic."

Dr. Lea felt that she had recovered from her failure to remember the delightful patient right away. She had already violated one of her own rules of always looking up hospital records on new clinic patient appointments beforehand. *Not doing that again,* she resolved to herself.

Dr. Lea recalled Pearl quite clearly now that she had made the connection. Pearl had indeed been quite sick in the hospital when she'd met her that time, probably four to six months ago, she estimated. *No wonder I didn't recognize her; she was in the ICU for sepsis and bacteremic shock and was severely anemic, if I recall correctly. I believe her hemoglobin was 4.6, barely a third or quarter of the normal amount.*

I'm surprised she looks so good today; the pallor is gone, and she's bright and cheery. She has makeup on with rosy cheeks; bright red, almost garish lipstick; and neatly coiffed hair, with just a hint of red. I'm sure her hair was much redder when she was young, much like my mom's. Her matching purse and shoes are too much. What is it about her? Already I feel like I haven't met anyone quite like her before.

"No worries, doctor. I'm surprised you remember me at all. You've seen so many patients, and you were caught off guard." Pearl clearly believed this. *Oh, this young doctor needs to go easy on herself.*

"Thank you, Pearl. Do you understand why you're seeing me today?"

"Yes, doctor. I'm seeing you today to help with my symptoms. That's what palliative care does, right? That's what I remember anyway from how it was explained to me at the hospital."

"Correct. Do you have any questions about palliative care? About what it is or what it isn't?"

"All I remember is that you're an expert in treating symptoms. Is there more to it than that? I'm afraid I didn't read the brochure the hospital discharge planner gave me." *I'm embarrassed; I should have read that before coming into the office. That one's on me; we're even.*

"Glad to clarify for you. Symptom management is the majority of what I do, but our team does much more than that. As part of our comprehensive palliative care team, we have a nurse case manager for you, a social worker, and then there's a group of doctors and nurse practitioners I work with. Sometimes we work in the hospital and also rotate outside the hospital for outpatient visits. I was appointed to start outside, primarily in the clinic, and to do house calls too.

"This team will help you with your symptoms for sure and then with other needs that may come up while you're getting your treatments. To be clear, we are not your cancer team but work together with them to help you feel as well as possible. For your symptoms related to your cancer and treatment, we'll go to your team. We're on call twenty-four hours a day and will handle prescribing medications to help with pain, nausea, constipation, trouble sleeping, et cetera."

"But you aren't my primary care doctor, right?"

"Correct again. We are not your primary care doctor. You will still go to them or contact them for your other health concerns, such as if you have high blood pressure, arthritis, or diabetes, for example."

"Got it."

"Furthermore, we can help with your advance directives or power of attorney for health care completion. Are you familiar with this terminology? Do you have one completed already? Our records don't show one."

"Hmmm. Let me think. Is that where I've picked out my casket and who gets my money and belongings after I die?"

"No, that's different. Those financial matters are handled

by you telling your family what you want to leave or donate to people, like an inheritance. Those wishes may be written and documented in a will or a trust. Many times the advance directive document is completed at the same time if you work through an attorney.

The advance directive or power of attorney is a document in which you designate your decision-maker if you can't medically make decisions, along with your wishes for treatment. Does that ring a bell?"

"Yes, yes, that's it. I don't remember anything about the power of attorney papers you mentioned, though. I'll have to look at home in my file."

"Yes, do that, and if you find it be sure to bring the advance directive back with you next time so we can be sure it's accurate and the way you want it to read. You can change your mind with regard to these documents and update them legally, but it has to be done properly. Our social worker, Robert, will give you a phone call in a week or two, if that's okay with you, to check and see how that's going. He can also help you complete one or get you started with the proper forms. You don't have to have an attorney draw it up for you—unless, of course, that's how you want to do it. Maybe if it's necessary you can work with him to update your other legal documents."

Pearl nodded in understanding but was looking past the doctor somewhat blankly.

"Are you okay, Pearl?" the doctor asked, noting tears welling up in Pearl's eyes. She reached over to the counter for the tissue box, but Pearl was already in her purse pulling one out.

"I'll be fine. Just give me a minute. This conversation is reminding me of when my husband died suddenly, and we didn't have time to talk this stuff over. It was so difficult without knowing what he wanted. That's what made me do it for my-self and my family. It's good to know it can be changed; there have been some things going on in my family that make me question my previous ideas."

"So, you do have one, then? I thought you said . . ."

"Oh, I recall it now. I just needed a bit of a nudge to re-member." Pearl finished dabbing her eyes and placed the tissue back in her purse. *Oh, Patrick.*

"What else shall we cover today?" Pearl asked, gathering herself.

"Tell me what you understand is going on with your active cancer," Dr. Lea prompted, her pen poised above the notepaper.

"Well, as I understand it, I have a type of chronic leukemia that's secondary to my treatment for breast cancer more than twenty years ago. I went through a stem cell transplant for it and took a type of chemo they called TKI. Neither one worked well for me, unfortunately."

"How does that make you feel?" Dr. Lea asked.

"You mean from the transplant and the TKI or how do I feel about it not working?"

"Yes, I meant about how you feel regarding the transplant and the treatment not working."

"Well, I'm disappointed. I hoped that at my age of 76 I might get results and have more time, but I'm not crying about it if that's what you mean. The transplant was a lot to go through, but I had high hopes from it. The TKI didn't bother me too much, other than fatigue. I took a couple short naps a day—but not every day, mind you."

"Your notes from your cancer doctor say you're still taking the TKI. It's called Tykitrol here in the US. He says in his notes that you may get some long-term benefits from staying on it, although that is not for sure based on the medical research.

He said you will talk it over at your next visit with him. Besides the fatigue, any other side effects from it?"

"Not that I know."

"Okay, that's good. We can talk more about it on your future visits with me. How did they find out it wasn't working?"

"I guess when I had my abdominal scans it showed enlarging lymph nodes, and the cancer doctor told me that was causing the vague ache I have in my sides and back."

"Yes, I have to agree with that based on your scan results and the symptoms you're having. I want to switch gears a little bit and come back to your pain. With all that you went through for your breast cancer and now ending up with the chronic myeloid leukemia, do you regret your breast cancer treatment?"

"No, not at all. I got so many good years from the treatment that getting this now doesn't make me look back and with any regret. Very much the opposite. I was grateful for the years it gave me, and I felt so good!"

"Thanks. I just wanted to be sure to give you a chance to let me know. Now, tell me more about your pain. What does it feel like? Where do you feel it? What makes it feel better or worse?"

"Sure. The pain is like a strong ache at its worst. In both sides." Pearl rubbed both of her sides with her hands to indicate the location. She had already done that three times that Dr. Lea had noticed. "It isn't one small spot but a general area. It's definitely worse at night but less during the day, and it doesn't seem to matter what I'm doing to cause it or make it stronger. A pain pill helps, but I only take it at night when it bothers me the most."

"So, the medicine does help, and it's enough for you?" *This is now the fourth time Pearl has rubbed her sides.*

"Oh, yes."

"We'll stick with that medicine for your pain, then. Your bowel and bladder control and habits are working fine?"

"Yes." *This doctor is going over everything.*

"Do you have other areas of pain?"

"No."

"Other stomach related symptoms, such as nausea or vomiting? Any trouble with breathing or coughing?"

"No, none I've noticed for any of that."

"What about bruising easily? Or bleeding from your gums or nose?" *I hope she isn't getting tired of the questions. As my trainers told me, investing in the doctor-patient relationship early on with more time and effort helps in the long run by establishing a good foundation to rely on in case it gets more difficult to communicate later on.*

"It's maybe a little easier to bruise, and occasionally my gums bleed, but not much or often. If you hadn't mentioned it I wouldn't have recalled it."

Through the rest of the first visit, additional review of her medical history included more details about her breast cancer. She had been treated at the time with breast removal surgery, plus additional radiation therapy to the area and adjuvant chemotherapy to lessen the chance of any recurrence. There had been none over the years, and Pearl had remained on a preventive hormone blocker.

She had developed the CML within the last five years; it's a chronic form of leukemia that sometimes develops after previous cancer treatment. It was felt that her chromosome-analysis-detected Philadelphia chromosome had made her more susceptible to the CML from her chemotherapy, and her genetic profile indicated an intermediate to high-risk for progression. She tolerated only Tykitrol of the TKIs available.

Her clinical physical exam by Dr. Lea found nothing un-expected: normal vital signs; a few superficial bruises on her forearms and hand dorsum but none on her mucus membranes, which were of a normal pink color; lungs clear to all fields and all the way to the bases; and heart tones crisp with normal sounding S_1 and S_2 (the *lub-dub* of normal heart sounds heard with the stethoscope), with no murmurs, clicks, or rubs. Her abdomen had palpable fullness in the flanks, and there was a suggestion of fullness under the rib margin on the left consis-tent with mild splenomegaly, but the liver was normal, as were the bowel sounds. No peripheral edema. A neuro exam was not conducted except to note that there were no tremors and that the patient presented with normal speech and normal thought content and pattern. A normal gait and balance were noted.

"Pearl, do you have any questions for me? I've asked a lot of them today, but it's all to get to know you better and help me take care of you. I hope that's okay."

"Yes, that's absolutely fine. Thank you. How do you think I'm doing? Should I do anything different?"

"I will be watching your course of illness and paying at-tention to your symptoms, especially your pain. We can also talk about your disease as we go along. Palliative care focuses on your goals for your health and makes sure your medical care matches those goals; this is the simplest definition of palliative care I can offer. We are on your team and will take good care of you."

"I know you will. I'm confident of that. When do I see you again, Dr. Lea?"

"Let's meet again in six weeks, right here at the cancer clinic."

Later, while Dr. Lea charted on Pearl's record, she noticed in the oncology notes that there was a downward trending weight and that the pain medication had been added a few months earlier. *I will be sure to keep watch on this. It's remarkable how well she's tolerating her TKI, and she accepts her condition so well. I don't know what she has been told about prognosis—we'll talk more about that next time.*

Pearl's past medical history also included mild adult-onset diabetes mellitus, which was treated only with diet, and she was off her blood pressure medication with good blood pressure readings. She was a retired elementary school teacher, widowed for several years and with a son and daughter, both living nearby.

Dr. Lea finished the charting and found herself smiling, uncertain why or if she should. *For some reason I believe Pearl is going to be a different kind of patient for me.*

2

PEARL

PAIN 1

Six Weeks Later

"KNOCK, knock. Anybody home?" Dr. Lea greeted Pearl, entering the clinic room on their next visit together.

"Good morning, Dr. Lea," Pearl replied.

"How are you doing?"

"About the same."

"How's your pain?" *Well, she's not offering much in the way of expanding on her symptoms, so I'll drill down into it more.* "What I want to know is if you still have the same amount of pain. I didn't have you rate it last time. You probably know the routine of giving it a score from 0 to 10, with 10 being the worst pain you can imagine and 0 being none."

"When I have pain, I'd give it a 2 or 3 at the worst. Same place," as Pearl rubbed her sides after setting her purse down on the floor next to her chair.

"Does the hydrocodone/acetaminophen combination give you relief? Last time you told me you took it only at nighttime."

"Right. It's all still the same. No trouble with the medicine, and I'm taking something to keep my bowels moving regularly. No other troubles."

"That's all good. How is your TKI working for you? Have you had more scans yet?"

"No scans, but one is scheduled for two weeks from now." Pearl double-checked on the calendar she pulled out of her purse.

"Okay. Thanks. I didn't see any results of testing show up. How are you feeling about the test coming up? Are you getting nervous about the results?"

"Not too much. I try not to think about it. I keep busy and positive."

Dr. Lea jots a note to follow up on that. *Pearl is not letting on, but it's bothering her more than she wants to tell me.*

"Let's talk about your advance directive, the power of attorney for health care. You found it okay? How was your conversation with Robert, the social worker?"

"Yes, it was in my file. It's several years old, though. Robert called. We spoke briefly about it. I told him I was going to work on it."

"And did you?"

"No, not really. I mean, I pulled it out, and it's sitting on my dining room table; it doubles as my desk these days. My daughter noticed it when she was over; I saw her eyes glance down at it, but she didn't say anything, and neither did I."

"It's important to keep working on it. The advance directive is like a road map or atlas. Have you ever used Triple A, the American Automobile Association?" Pearl nodded. "You'll probably recall, then, that they provide a printed-out map of your vacation route, with page-by-page turns. They do this in great detail so you won't get lost or make a wrong turn and so you can have confidence you will arrive at your destination. That's what the advance directive is for you, your family, and your health care providers. It gives detailed guidance—directions just like a map—for the kind of care you want for yourself. In this way you'll get the care you want that matches your health care wishes.

"Most importantly, it specifies the person or persons you want to make decisions for you if you're unable to do this. In our society and culture, autonomy—that is, making your own decisions—is considered very important and is highly valued. Having the advance directive maps out for those caring for you the steps you want or maybe some things you don't want to have done."

Pearl nods, slowly this time, and with that faraway look again. *Dr. Lea is right about this. I know it makes sense, obviously, but it's just too difficult to think or talk about. I don't want to sadden my family.*

"Pearl, am I getting through to you?" Dr. Lea asked. She tried to make eye contact with her patient, but a longer pause ensued with Pearl not breaking her faraway gaze. *No tears this time.*

Dr. Lea continued, "In another sense it's like a final gift to your family so they don't have to wonder what you would decide. It can give them peace of mind on these kinds of decisions when their emotions in the moment can be strong and even misleading them or causing conflict and disagreement among them. The person you choose to be your decision-maker must be someone you trust to make sure the plan—or map, as you might think of it, going back to our Triple A analogy—is followed according to your wishes and hopes.

"Having this road map gives clear guidance, allows your medical care to be in line with your desires, and avoids unnecessary delays in decision-making for the care you might need. And it gives you peace of mind." *Still no tears, and I like the way she's now looking right at me as I wrap this up.*

"One more thing, before I stop here and examine you. Sometimes people believe that talking about these matters will bring these issues on them sooner, physically. Let me tell you that in my experience so far that's simply not true. Most people feel relieved to have the talking behind them and the decisions settled. Then they don't have to dwell on those issues until or if further action is needed. Pearl, what are you thinking?"

"Dr. Lea, you are absolutely right; you're a thousand times right. The sadness of the past is miring me down and keeping me from moving forward. I want to be mobile, not stuck. You've made me realize this. Yes, I completed one of those documents years ago, but what I wrote down then isn't what I really want now—not at all. You've helped me realize that the pain of the past can hinder me now. I don't want that."

Pearl is getting it, truly getting it. "I know I was quite direct with you, but I believed it was necessary to get across the key points. I had a sense you were stuck, as you said."

"Have Robert call me in a couple weeks. This time I'll talk with him. Next time you'll see progress, doctor."

"Glad to have a breakthrough with you on this tough subject. Now, back to your physical pain. Do you need a prescription for the pain medication? If not now, at any time you can call our number and request some. Is there anything else?"

"No, I don't think so. See you again in six weeks?"

"Yes, go ahead and set it up on your way out of the clinic, but before you leave I want to listen to your heart and lungs, feel your abdomen, and look for edema and bruising." Dr. Lea went through her exam as she had done at the previous visit, noting no changes. She stood back from the exam table.

Pearl asked, "Dr. Lea, are you a hugging person? I want to give you a hug to show my appreciation of your efforts for me."

"Sure, Pearl, I'm fine with that." A brief hug and goodbyes ensued.

3

PEARL

PALLIATIVE CARE SUMMARY 1

COVERED early in the story is an explanation of palliative care. For our discussion, consider palliative care to be a medical specialty or service that:

1. Works with patients experiencing serious illness and its burden.

2. Is attentive to symptom relief for the whole person, whether it is physical, emotional, social, or spiritual distress from the serious illness.

3. Helps and leads the patient to determine and then follow directions in order to reach their health care goals to achieve their desired quality of life.

In its most fundamental definition, palliative care is simply the medical care of a patient with a serious illness, focusing on their goals for their care. Many patients wrongly believe that palliative care means that the medical personnel are giving up on them. I've heard patients say things like "You're all giving up on me," "I have more fight in me," or "I don't want to give up." Instead of these kinds of responses, consider palliative care as more about making sure their care goals are pursued or met so they can reach the quality of life they hope for. This type of care is not at all about giving up but about being absolutely certain—about making sure.

The term "palliative" is derived from the Latin term for "to palliate," which means "to cloak" (*pallium*). The more modern use of the term is "to conceal" or "to hide." It was first used in the fifteenth century when a cloak was worn by educators and philosophers. Palliative care is a type of medical care offered to provide a layer of comfort and thus lessen the severity of the symptoms of the disease or the effects of treatment. Palliative care does not intend to treat the underlying condition; that responsibility lies with the treating medical team of the patient's primary care provider or specialist. Think of it in terms of a cloak of protection and comfort that covers the patient in their journey.

A discussion about goals of care helps the provider discover what the patient desires for their health care. This means figuring out the balance between the two possible avenues of care that will give them an acceptable quality of life (to move forward with a given treatment or forego it). Just because a treatment is "out there" or available doesn't mean it is right for every individual. The patient must weigh the pros and cons and decide whether or not to go through with the available treatment.

You can see how important these goals of care discussions become when the care providers are sorting through options or alternatives. There must be clear information sharing, complete understanding of the alternatives and prognoses, and correct application of the chosen course of action in terms of the patient's medical situation. The palliative care team can lead the way in these discussions because of their expertise and experience, and they can help share the results of the discussions and their observations with the rest of the health care team.

Finding the appropriate timing of a palliative care referral can be tricky to sort out, but it mainly depends on the acute severity of the patient's serious illness and how it is affecting their functional status. Functional status refers to a formal or informal evaluation of how well a patient can perform everyday tasks. These daily activities include walking and balancing; doing household chores; driving; staying safe at home; communicating; preparing meals; managing bathroom needs and personal hygiene; bathing; and taking care of their medical needs, including medications.

Most of the time that timing decision is based more on a general feeling or sense by the medical team members than on a formal testing process. The testing can be more formal when it relates to checking someone's mental health or physical skills, such as strength, walking ability, or balance; administering a driver's assessment test; or determining whether an alternative placement might be necessary.

There are no specific rules for when to refer someone for palliative care, but there are situations when making a referral is a good idea. The patient often shows signs that their advanced serious illness or condition is getting worse; this is referred to as progression. While progression is very common after cancer diagnoses, any advancing serious illness can qualify.

Some common examples include severe kidney failure, heart failure, and chronic lung problems like emphysema and chronic bronchitis with advanced symptoms. Liver diseases can also be a reason for referral, as can neurological conditions such as worsening dementia, severe stroke, or Parkinson's disease. This is not a complete list, but it does include some of the more common situations. The urgency of the referral depends on how acutely severe ("suddenly changing") the person's condition is, especially if there are or could be serious and life-threatening complications or consequences.

In a long-term situation palliative care also relates to how quickly the disease is worsening, since progression can cause distressing symptoms for the patient. Another scenario that might lead to a palliative care referral is when a patient visits the emergency department multiple times in a short time frame for an ongoing advanced serious illness.

This last option for a referral mentioned above doesn't occur very often; patients with serious illness typically come back to the emergency room multiple times before they are referred. This doesn't mean that the hospital staff has forgotten about the palliative care option, but patients often have many reasons for not wanting to accept palliative care. Similarly, if a patient goes to their primary care doctor or specialist repeatedly for the same advanced illness, this is also a reason to refer them to palliative care.

Hopefully the information in this book will help patients to better understand palliative care and will encourage them to ask for a referral to it.

Examples of cases referred for palliative care

CHF or other advanced heart disease
COPD with advanced symptoms and chronic respiratory failure
Advanced kidney failure
Acute or chronic stroke with complications
Parkinson's disease with advanced or poorly controlled symptoms

Alzheimer's or similar dementia with progressive disease
Advanced stages of cancer
Repeat hospitalizations for same advanced condition
Repeat or multiple emergency department visits for same advanced condition
Repeat of multiple office visits for same advanced condition

If someone's health gets worse because of any of the illnesses or disorders mentioned in the chart, or if their overall health declines, palliative care should be considered. The overall decline is seen when there is a decrease in function, which can include sudden or unexpected weight loss, weakness, tiredness, doing less, trouble moving around, or worsening symptoms from their advanced serious illness. An example is having more trouble breathing because of heart or lung disease.

———

A patient's palliative care team members are experts in talking about these serious illnesses and conditions. Think of the palliative care consultation as a way to better understand the person's condition and outlook.

Palliative care programs are available both in hospitals and outside the hospital at other locations, such as in clinics. Currently, more than 80 percent of medium and larger hospitals have a program for inpatient palliative care.[3] These are excellent at helping patients and their families understand complicated medical issues. The team members discuss care goals, as mentioned above, and help manage symptoms in the hospital to make the patient feel comfortable. They can help with symptoms like pain, trouble breathing, feeling nausea, and vomiting. The palliative care (commonly shortened to PC) team can help in any area of the hospital, extending from the emergency department to the intensive care unit to the medical/surgical floors.

In certain special situations there are teams trained in pediatric palliative care that can assist in children's hospital areas, including the emergency department, critical care units, medical-surgical units, or high-risk obstetrical units.

What is less certain is whether there are palliative care programs available in the patient's community for outpatient services. The hospital palliative care team will know about community palliative care programs and might suggest follow up care. The primary care doctor's office can also help find and refer the patient to these services. Online resources such as getpalliativecare.org can help find programs in a patient's community.

———

Advance directives are extremely important for knowing what kind of medical care a patient wants and what their goals are. They are like a road map outlining the directions and turns for arriving at a destination. There might be changes to the documents at any time based on what happens along the route. These documents are meant to be changed if needed.

Another important point is that, although finishing the document is important, it isn't the final answer in every case. It is preferred to have the document completed, but the conversation regarding what it contains or will contain is most important. It is best to have the directives written down legally because they will then be recognized in all situations and followed appropriately and confidently by the medical team caring for the patient.

Spelling out the desires and goals ahead of time makes a confusing situation easier to understand and navigate. The hospital team can provide care effectively instead of wasting time waiting for the family or other decision makers to clarify the preferences or resolve conflicts. This decision is important because it should align with the goals and wishes of the patient. When a legal form is filled out clearly stating these wishes, it can be followed instead of guessed at.

The advance directive can be written in a formal or informal way and can be specific or general. Just remember that having something in writing is better than having nothing. The designated decision-maker, sometimes called the surrogate or agent, is the person chosen ahead of time who best knows the patient's wishes and can guide the medical team correctly. Having the choices written out leaves no questions about who should make decisions or clarify what the patient wants for their medical care.

Following is my own list of the top ten reasons to complete an advance directive. It lists these reasons from least to most important, similar to the way David Letterman used to present his Top Ten lists.

My Top 10 Reasons for Advance Care Planning

10. Makes your attorney happy

9. Resolves Conflict

8. Better Care

7. Conversation Starter

6. Sets an Example

5. Gives a Clear Direction

4. Burden Relief

3. Treated the Way You Want to Be

2. Makes Sure

1. Peace of Mind

The advance directive can be a separate, stand-alone document or included with other estate planning papers created by a lawyer. If the stand-alone option is preferred, the patient can draft the directive on their own or with a lawyer. If they decide to do it on their own, the important steps are to appoint the decision-maker and to obtain the necessary signatures, including those of witnesses.

To be eligible the witnesses cannot be the patient's relatives and cannot stand to receive any inheritance or benefits from the patient. A witness must be an adult of "sound mind." It is important to understand the rules of the state in which one lives. A witness cannot be the same person the patient chooses to make decisions.

Remember that healthcare workers are not always allowed to be witnesses. Some states require a witness to be a notary, but this rule is not universal, and the situation can vary from state to state or even within different areas of the same state. The agent or decision-maker also needs to sign the form to take on the responsibility.

The number of details and choices about medical care in the advance directive are completely at the discretion of the person making the decisions. The wording can be very specific or general but should include enough details to help the agent make good decisions. The patient or decision-maker can use forms that designate pre-written choices or write out their wishes in their own language. Both options are fine. An important part of determining and revealing one's choices and plans entails the patient talking with important people in their life. At the very least, in the absence of a completed document, the decision-maker should know about the patient's choices.

When looking at the medical information in the document or while discussing care goals, the decision-maker or patient should think about what matters to them. Many times it comes down to a preference for either a better quality of life or a longer life. The palliative care team can assist with this review and discussion, together with advice from the patient's primary care doctor and other specialists. Each individual is unique, and objective and skilled professionals can help guide and focus the conversation, especially in complicated situations.

It is helpful to bear in mind that each individual patient carries influences from their own past or family experiences, their understanding of their condition, their awareness of how it affects their life and daily functioning, and sometimes even their prognosis. The person needs to think about that delicate balance between quality and quantity of life. This is about asking whether the potential treatment or intervention or procedure to gain longer life is worth the cost in terms of its likely effect on the quality of life. There are no right or wrong answers, but figuring this out can be hard. It is best to do this reflecting when not in a crisis mode, if possible.

The completed advance directive forms should not be kept at home in a safe or safety deposit box; they are meant to be shared. Copies are just as good as the original, and the patient should keep one for himself or herself, their chosen decision-maker (the surrogate or agent), at their doctor's office, and with the hospital or healthcare system. When the information is added to the hospital's electronic records the patient's medical providers can access it whenever they need to.

When the person's wishes and goals are clearly written down, research shows that patients receive better care, family conflicts over these issues can be resolved, and it is easier for the family to make tough emotional decisions. Taking this step early on also provides clear and simple directions for the medical team, allowing them to provide the care the patient wants and needs in a timely and efficient manner. Ultimately, this gives all involved peace of mind in the knowledge that the big decisions have been handled.

The individual can always decide to let others make these decisions, even if they are able to make them themselves. The patient can take back (revoke) the document or change what it says at any time, as long as they understand what they are doing (they must still have the necessary competency to make changes to the document).

For more information on advance directives and decision-making ability, see the Appendix.

How can one get help for completing their advance directives? A community has many resources, as well as information available online and in books. The two most common options, however, are to go to their attorney or doctor's office to get the process started. Many palliative care programs have a social worker on their team who can help the person complete the form or offer guidance through their power of attorney documents.

Some communities have a "Senior Services" clearinghouse that offers free counseling and/or helps with the advance directive. If the patient opts to pursue this on their own, it is imperative that they pay attention to the rules for the state they live in. The rules and regulations can be different in each state, so what applies in one state might not be valid in another. If the person moves out of state, they should make sure to educate themselves on any changes they must make to comply with the new state's regulations.

An advance directive is not a will, a living will, or a funeral plan. These are different documents for planning. I have had patients tell me that one of these is their advance directive; this is a common misunderstanding.

Another term used for an advance directive is Power of Attorney for Health Care, sometimes with the word "Durable" at the front of the title. These refer to the exact same document.

If the person has filled out an advance directive, they are among the approximately 30 percent of Americans who have done so. If they haven't finished one yet, they are only an hour or so away from getting it done. First, the patient should make sure that they have chosen a surrogate or agent (decision-maker)—the most important step—and have secured their permission to take on this responsibility.

To reiterate, they should remember that advance directives can always be changed if they change their mind or further developments in their life require a review of the document. The added changes might include specific details on the desired medical care following more thorough discussion or thought on the matter and once the patient has been fully informed about their medical conditions.

4

PEARL

TALK TURKEY

Six Weeks Later

"Yes, Dr. Lea, I did speak with Robert. He was helpful. I found my previous power of attorney document, and we reviewed it together. All the signatures were proper, he said, so it's legitimate. At least for now I've made no changes, but I'm thinking more and more about doing some things differently."

"That's terrific news, Pearl. So glad to hear you're working on it. Do you have a plan for that?"

"Yes, I do. I'm calling it Talking Turkey. With the Thanksgiving holiday coming up and family gathering at my home, I thought it might be a good time to spring this issue on my kids and talk more about it."

"Great idea. That would be a very good time for it. You could introduce it creatively to them. Maybe try an approach like, 'At this Thanksgiving we aren't only going to eat turkey but talk turkey too. Gobble, gobble." Both chuckled.

"And I'll flap my arms like wings when I do it!" Pearl demonstrated her arm motions. "They'll get a kick out of that!"

"It's good to have fun along with your serious stuff—if it fits into your family dynamic."

"Oh, that's no problem. We're all crazier than bed bugs."

"Well, enjoy." Dr. Lea then moved the conversation forward. "Tell me about your pain. How is it doing? Have you changed how much pain medicine you're needing to take, other than at bedtime?"

"So far, no. It's working for me. I would say the pain is basically about the same." Pearl rubbed her sides absently.

"Okay, that's fine then. You'll tell me when it changes, right?"

"For sure I will, Dr. Lea." Pearl looked down momentarily and then asked, "What else do you want to know about?"

"Any other new symptoms? Wat about your test results?"

"No other new symptoms. The results show the large abdominal lymph nodes are the same—or slightly larger in one of them."

"Are you still taking the Tykitrol?"

"Yes, same dose. No changes. And yes, I'm still tired during the daytime, but so far it doesn't stop me from doing what I want." *I knew she was going to ask me about the fatigue, so I just went ahead and told her. Not sure I want to tell her I'm afraid to stop the Tykitrol at this point. There she is, tapping her cheek.*

"Okay, right. It appears you're satisfied with staying on it." *Hmmm. I wish I knew for sure she's telling me straight about the fatigue not giving her more trouble. I think she'll tell me when it's time for me to know. I hope she trusts me.* Dr. Lea tapped on her laptop screen to review the abdominal imaging results herself and then sat for a moment silently mulling over them.

After finishing her review of the scan results, Dr. Lea asked, "Pearl, do you need any prescriptions from me today?"

"No. I called in just over a week ago for the pain medication, and you and your team took care of it for me right away. I still take the other bowel regimen, and it keeps me regular."

"That's all good. Well, if there isn't anything else, we'll get you on your way. What's next for you this morning?"

"Going to get my hair done. It's the third Thursday of the month, so it's my hairdresser day."

"Well, good. Let's space your next appointment out a little bit longer since there haven't been any changes since we began seeing you. Let's make it two or three months. Are you okay with that, Pearl?"

"Yes, that's fine. Two months. Thanks, Dr. Lea."

"Goodbye, Pearl." *No hugs this time.*

5

PEARL

PAIN – 2

Two Months Later

"PEARL, good to see you." Dr. Lea shook hands with Pearl this time. "It's been two months since your last visit and five months since we began seeing you. And you haven't been back to the hospital."

"You're right. Isn't that great!"

"I believe so too. How did your Thanksgiving go with your family and the talking turkey, as you put it last time?"

"Overall, I was pleased with how it went. Besides the food turning out well, the conversations were full and meaningful. My son and daughter both appreciated the talk. It was better than I expected—I don't know why it went so well, but it did. I was expecting some pushback or disagreement. They do argue still even as adults, and the two of them don't see eye-to-eye on many things, but this time it was almost perfect."

"Well, that sounds like a pleasant surprise. Makes for a better holiday too. So, having the tough conversation didn't spoil the day?"

"No, not at all."

"Well, maybe it happened that way because you took a positive approach, and they can see you're doing okay at this point."

"Maybe so." Pearl hesitated. "Or maybe it was the custard pie!"

"Custard pie—not pumpkin pie?"

"Yes, it's an old Irish family recipe. We have it on birthdays and Thanksgiving."

"It sounds delicious. Are you done with the advance directive changes? Did you write them out? And what about your decision-maker?"

"I have written it out, and I'm going to change my decision-maker from my son, who is the older one, to my daughter, as I think she's more in tune with what I'm thinking and willing to follow my wishes. Not sure how my son will take that, but I'm fairly sure that's what I'm going to do. I've written out my DNR decision—I think that's what it's called—and some other medical procedures I don't want any longer."

"You seem sure about it. That's good. Do you need any further help or information from me or the social worker?"

"No, not at this point. Maybe before I finalize it. I'll keep it in mind." *I wonder if I should tell her about my experience with my husband's story and the power of attorney—or, really, the lack of it? Maybe if she waits a few seconds longer, then I'll . . .*

"Pearl, tell me about your pain. Any changes in severity, location, or timing, and then, how effective is your pain medicine?"

"There has been a change, slight but definite." Pearl rubbed her sides in her customary way. "It's beginning to hurt more in the morning when I wake up, even if—or I mean *when*—I take my pain medicine at bedtime. It feels like it's in the same location but a little stronger. I'm still able to do what I want in the daytime, but I'll have to say it aches more."

"I see—that is a change." *This time she kept rubbing her sides through the whole time she talked about the pain. That's a change too.* "Well, let's talk more about your pain medicine. You're taking one or two tabs at bedtime?"

"One."

"Do you have to take any more in the morning when it's still achy? And how strong is the pain in the morning?"

"I've thought about taking another one in the morning but haven't tried it yet. Yes, the pain at night is a three or four, and in the morning it's a two or three, when before I had none."

"Any trouble with your urine control?"

"No, and I'm still doing the bowel regimen. That's working fine too."

"Pearl, what if we try having you take a morning medicine for your pain if it's a three? And for milder achy pain in the morning let's have you try the acetaminophen only, not the strong combination medicine. Take at least 500 mg. of the acetaminophen—that's one tablet—and you can take two at a time if needed for a pain level of three or higher. I know you said the pain isn't interfering with your activities, but staying ahead of it is good to do. We won't look at changing your strong pain medicine at this time unless it isn't able to control it or you have trouble with it. And keep in mind not to take more than four of the extra-strength acetaminophens per day. We need to watch your total for the day, as there's acetaminophen in your strong pain tablet too."

"Got it, Dr. Lea. I like this approach." *I like her; she listens to me and isn't overly aggressive with changing my medications around.*

"That's our plan, then. Tell me what oncology has said about your continuation on Tykitrol? And how is your fatigue?"

"Yes, still on it. They said last time that with the slight increase in the size of my abdominal lymph nodes it's still up to me whether I continue it. They agree with me either way I decide."

"Okay, then. When you're interested in talking about it more, you can mention it to your oncologist, or we can give you some guidance. How is your fatigue?"

"Thanks, I'll do that. For now I want to take it. The fatigue isn't a problem. I'm used to it and adjust what I do to deal with it."

Dr. Lea completed her exam of Pearl, observing no changes from her previous visit. The lymph nodes on the scan were too deep in the abdomen to be able to feel them by a physical exam.

"Okay. Well, that wraps up our visit. Let's have you back in two to three months. We'll have our nurse call you in a couple weeks to check on your pain and the medicine for it. If you need something before then, you can call us and move up your appointment. And you'll be having another scan by then."

"Right. That all sounds good to me. I'll set it up on my way out."

"Thanks, Pearl." *Again, no hug this time.*

6

PEARL

PALLIATIVE CARE SUMMARY – 2

WE'VE seen that the advance directive completion is a process involving more than getting a document completed, signed, and witnessed. For the patient it entails talking with people who are important in their life, whether or not they are in the family. The designation of one's decision-maker (agent or surrogate) is the most important decision step. It is often the person in the family who is closest to the patient. However, sometimes that is impossible or impractical.

It is wise for the patient to think about and discuss their options for who to choose before a crisis or an urgent situation arises. Yet again, it's important to bear in mind that changes are always possible and that the patient should take the time to think about and talk this over with concerned parties. Speaking with their doctor is helpful, since the physician can provide key information about the medical circumstances that might be encountered that will require decisions.

The palliative care team can help the patient prepare for these situations as well. A strong feature of the staff's experience is foreseeing what situations and decisions may lie ahead. Examples of such decisions might include use of a feeding tube, appropriate bridge treatment for conditions such as advanced dementia or cancer, cancer-related treatment complications, or the best course of action related to a sudden acute illness like a stroke or traumatic injury. Each of these situations calls for a different perspective and discussion of unique details concerning the patient's medical conditions or abilities. It's all about how the patient is feeling and functioning. The palliative care team is experienced and poised to help with sorting through the complexities. They can help start discussions or make decisions.

Other complex examples include the patient's DNAR (Do Not Attempt Resuscitation) status and the advisability of proposed surgeries—not just for cancer, for example, but also for the individual's advanced dementia. The situation may also involve figuring out how a patient's weakness or frailty will affect medical treatment and predicting outcomes to facilitate treatment decisions. This point applies not only to cancer but also to other treatments that can affect how long a patient might live.

Further examples are dialysis for failing kidneys during an advanced serious illness and getting a second opinion from other specialists or specialized care centers. The palliative care approach aims to provide the patient and their loved ones with honest and realistic information based on the patient's condition, ability to function, and expected prognosis. The interaction of these three factors—patient condition, function, and prognosis—along with guidance from the advance directive, can help decide the best path to take.

If you find yourself or someone close to you in this situation, it makes sense to ask for a referral to palliative care if one hasn't already been offered. Most medium-to-large community hospitals or referral centers have staff available to assist with a referral, and most of these individuals work in the hospital every day or are readily available to help. Even if they are asked to become involved later on during the course of the illness, they can be a helpful resource, experienced at going through extensive medical records and talking to doctors, primary care offices, specialists, and family members or caregivers to achieve a clear and informed understanding and assessment.

In addition, many medium sized or larger cities have outpatient palliative care teams that provide expert support outside of hospitals—although these are not as common. An online resource to find registered programs in one's area is getpalliativecare.org. This is a resource from a national palliative care organization called CAPC, Center to Advance Palliative Care. Asking for assistance from the patient's primary care office or hospital can also be a place to start. Another listing for palliative care in a given area can be found at PalliativeDoctors.org. This is a membership registry through the National Association for Palliative Care and Hospice Physicians.

Additionally, once hospice care has commenced, it is important to pay attention to the palliative care doctor's concern for the patient's quality of life, including how well symptoms are managed and how those symptoms affect their ability to live and function. The patient should be ready and willing to answer questions about how they are doing; their honest answers will help the providers in achieving the best quality of life for the patient and reaching care or treatment goals.

In the Appendix more topics are covered in which the palliative care team can be helpful for weighing the factors to reach decisions consistent with the patient's goals.

———

Pearl's story shows what can happen when people don't talk about their care goals. Pearl had experienced a difficult time with the way her husband had died because important issues hadn't been handled correctly or in a timely fashion, and this continued to affect her. She was not going through prolonged or complicated grief, but she did have a painful memory that lingered when she thought about it. Her daily life was not affected, as shown by her activities, but the difficult memory had caused her to be less open with the doctor. However, that experience had also been a profound lesson that ultimately inspired her to update her own advance directive.

Dr. Lea was a new physician who had graduated in the area of palliative care only a few months before she started seeing Pearl. She was still developing her style as an attending physician, though her confidence was growing with each patient encounter. Notice the way she would pause during a conversation with the patient, giving them time to think about what to say or to control their emotions. Dr. Lea didn't push Pearl to share her feelings or thoughts, even though they were clearly strong and deep seated. We can observe her planning her follow up for future encounters, built on the unfolding story.

Another advantage of palliative care is that it can be provided in different settings. So far, we've looked at visits in the hospital and clinics. However, the patient's home is in many cases the optimal setting. Think of "home" here as the place the patient feels most comfortable and least guarded; it might be a facility, for example. Visiting the patient in their own environment helps the clinical team, which includes not just doctors but also nurses, social workers, and chaplains.

Patients usually feel more relaxed at home, and the home visit allows the clinician to check the safety of the house or facility and learn more about the patient's lifestyle. This can provide important input with respect to their care and family interactions or for simply getting to know the patient better. When patients go to the clinic, on the other hand, the setting is inherently somewhat artificial. Sometimes the patient in the office or clinic will act in the way they think they should when seeing a doctor. Still, there are always those patients for whom the setting of the visit doesn't matter; they will remain true to themselves no matter where they are.

7

DALE

INTRODUCTIONS AND DEALS

First Home Visit

DR. Lea parked and picked up her stethoscope from the front seat of her car, along with her shoulder bag with her other medical tools and her tablet for AI charting, if Dale agreed to the technology. This would be her first time meeting Dale, but it wasn't Dale's first palliative care visit. He had been receiving outpatient palliative care for three years.

Dr. Lea enjoyed making house calls on Wednesdays. Seeing the patients in their own familiar environment provided information that could easily be missed in a clinic. In the home patients tend to feel less stress, and they don't have to face possible hurdles of transportation to and from the clinic. Seeing the patient in this more relaxed setting typically helps them talk more openly, which leads to a better and more accurate medical history.

The patient at home will probably not act as though they feel better or stronger than they really do, and this facilitates the provider receiving valuable insights. It's important to consider the home itself and its safety, especially for patients in palliative care who are living with at least one advanced serious illness. These patients often face weakness, fatigue, and a decline in their ability to function. The palliative care team had already noted all of this about Dale, since he had been receiving care for over three years, but it would be a good time to reassess these points when a new clinician arrived at the home.

It would depend on who one were to ask to determine whether Dale found the time useful or a waste. If Dale himself were taking the survey, his vote would be apparent. Dr. Lea had her tools and her experience, and she had looked through his medical records, especially the notes on palliative care from the doctor before her.

Dr. Marcus Dryden had retired from practicing medicine during the last year, and Dr. Lea had taken over his position. She would be the first to say that Dr. Dryden couldn't be replaced— especially not by a novice like herself. He had practiced for nearly thirty years in palliative care and hospice, with his first fifteen years as an emergency medicine physician. He had been instrumental in starting the palliative care fellowship and had handed it over twice after getting it going.

The first replacement had lasted for only two years because of the cold weather in the area—or so people thought. Dr. Dryden had felt obligated to lead the fellowship for six months longer before handing it over again, this time for good. The new physician was much more skilled and dedicated to teaching than the initial replacement doctor had been—not to mention that he was a seasoned Northerner. Dr. Dryden was glad to work in palliative care without having to lead the training program any longer.

Though no longer formally the program director, Dr. Dryden had continued teaching through lectures and had regularly overseen a mix of fellows, students, interns, and residents from different specialties.

Dr. Lea didn't even try to replace Dr. Dryden because that would have been impossible. She chose to be herself from the beginning and not to worry about anything else. She knew her predecessor because she had trained there, and she respected him. As a tribute to his excellent clinical skills and management of patients, she was grateful to encounter no need to make a lot of changes or to "clean up" any medical messes that might have been left behind.

Dale was one of Dr. Dryden's former patients. Although she and Dr. Dryden had never discussed this patient directly, and she had never met Dale before, she was prepared for this initial visit. The other staff, including the palliative care social worker and nurse, were aware of Dale's blunt and sometimes harsh way of speaking. However, he was usually very respectful when they visited his house or talked on the phone.

Dr. Lea had been counseled not to mind his sloppy appearance, although he wasn't expected to cause any problems during the visit. The nurse could not visit him today because she was at the palliative care clinic, and no one else on staff was available to accompany Dr. Lea for house calls on this particular day.

There were two cars in the cramped driveway, one of which clearly hadn't been driven in years. All four tires were flat, and the vehicle was covered in dirt and dust. Small twigs and leaves had blown in and were stuck in the wipers on the windshield and around the flat tires. Dr. Lea parked her modest Honda Accord behind the smaller, drivable Toyota Corolla. The rest of the front lawn looked maintained, though not perfectly, matching the appearance of the house.

Dale answered the door just as Dr. Lea finished her first knock.

"Come in, Doc. Don't mind the clutter—just rearranging furniture for the change in seasons. Not!"

"No problem. Are you Mr. Dale McComb?" Dr. Lea asked.

"Well, yes, that's me. Were you expecting to meet another Dale, like Dale Earnhardt, the race car driver? Or maybe King Tut in a flannel shirt?"

"No, I meant you, Mr. McComb—the one and only Mr. Dale McComb. I'm the one and only Dr. Lea Glendale. I took over some of Dr. Dryden's patients. He made sure I got his best ones!" Dr. Lea tried to seem slightly comedic to match Dale's tone; her response wasn't too smart-alecky or sidesplitting but tolerable for an initiation with Dale.

"Oh, you're a funny one, are you? We'll get along fine, as your nurse said we would. She bragged you up pretty good. Dr. Dryden—I liked him. Straight talker, no beating around the bush with him, and that's the way I like it. How about you, doc?"

"Same for me . . ." She was midsentence when he broke in.

"Call me, Dale. I'm Dale—have been my whole life. It's all I'll answer to anymore. The doc took care of my wife too. She died in hospice care two and a half years ago. God rest her soul." Dale put his hand over his heart and bowed briefly before rattling on, "Died right over there, on the couch. It was all of a sudden too. Everyone, including me, thought I would go first!"

He gestured across the room. It was dark in the living room, though it was the middle of the day. The only light was from an old floor lamp next to his recliner, but it barely enlightened the expansive room—possibly due to the thick layer of dust on the bulb and lampshade. His window shades were all down except in the dining area toward the back of the house, overlooking another area of ignored lawn with overgrown bushes and shade trees.

"Once Doc Dryden got here to see her, she was comfortable from then on. He made her feel rested too." Dale hobbled with his cane over to the recliner, "Doc, you have a seat; go ahead. Anywhere's fine," he swept his arm in an expansive gesturing covering the ample area. There were plenty of options, but the doctor settled on a hard kitchen chair. Then she noticed someone else in the kitchen.

"Hi, there. I'm Dr. Lea." She held out her hand as the person emerged into the room.

"Hi, I'm Hannah. I help Mr. Dale. I'm just tidying up the kitchen." She gave Dr. Lea a short and awkward handwave.

"Don't mind her, doc. Hannah's fine. I trust her."

"Thanks. Shall we get started, Dale?" Dr. Lea asked. She had her stethoscope around her neck already and her tablet opened.

"I don't mind if you use that recording thingamajig. Doc Dryden explained it to me and showed me how it works. I'm fine with it."

"Great, thanks. That'll make it easier for me. So, Dale, I've read through the notes from Dr. Dryden's last two visits and some of your medical records. But just so I can hear it from you, for what reasons were you referred to palliative care, and how is it going for you?"

"Well, as I recall it was because I went to the hospital emergency room too much. I couldn't catch my breath, and I used all my inhalers—my neb'lizers—and had oxygen on. Nothing helped, so I called the ambulance and went to the hospital, of course. It's what anyone else would do. Since Doc Dryden took that part over, I haven't been back to the hospital since.

Must be close to three years, I'd say. Pretty good track record." He started to shake a cigarette out of a pack but stopped as soon as it started to slide out.

"Haven't felt this good in years. Sure am glad he came along. I probably wouldn't be here if it weren't for Doc Dryden and the PC. That's what Doc and I called the kind of doctor he is— much easier for me to say than the other word, pally-or-other. He could say it fine, but not me." He smiled a little sheepishly.

"So, you had many episodes of feeling short of breath, would go to the hospital and get treatment there, they'd send you home, and then not too long after you'd have it happen all over again. That's right, then?"

"Yes, that's right—you've got it," Dale said.

"That's no way to live, back and forth like that. Did this come on over time, or did these episodes happen close together?"

"I'd say kind of both." He shook out the cigarette all the way and started to light up but stopped himself and set the lighter back down, still holding the unlit cigarette in his hand as if it were lit.

"Okay, I see. Did you go to see your family doctor after the hospital emergency visits?"

"Yes and no. Sometimes I did and sometimes I didn't. How's that for an answer, doc?"

"I get what you mean. How much are you smoking?"

"As much as I want."

"Dale," came the voice from the kitchen. "That's not the right way to talk to her."

"Oh, I suppose you're right," he hollered back. "Sorry, Doc, about that. I forget my manners once in a while, but I don't mean nothin' by it. Okay?"

"Yes, sure. We are getting to know each other in these early visits. I'm fine."

"See?!" Dale called out again toward the kitchen. A cabinet door shut a little harder right after he had said it.

"So, I will summarize some of your medical history, and you can correct me if I have something wrong. Your main medical problem is the COPD; that's the chronic lung disease from your smoking and from your decades of work in the foundry. Bad combination. You are 68 years old and have been disabled from the COPD since you were 59 years old. You still smoke, but it sounds like less than you did before. Have you quit before?"

"Oh, I've tried. Everyone begged me to quit. I tried the gum, the patch, and the pills—not all at once, you know." He smiled to himself at his joking retort. "My wife, all the doctors, and Doc Dryden too. He said even though I had advanced disease it would make a difference on how I feel, since my lungs were only working on about a third of what's normal, as he described it. So, I've tried. Shall I add you to the list too?"

"Yes, you might as well. I wouldn't be doing my job if I didn't tell you to quit due to how it harms you—besides the risks of the combination of oxygen and fires. I haven't seen an accident myself, but I've heard reliable stories of the dangers, and I don't want that to happen to you. By continuing to smoke you aren't helping yourself at all.

"Let's move on to your medications. You're taking your medications and your inhaler nebulizers as prescribed?"

"Yes, I sure am. Next?"

"Okay. The rest of your medication for cholesterol and some arthritis pain—you're taking those as prescribed?"

"Yup. Next? You're getting the hang of this, doc."

"I believe you're right. We are.

"Most people who have this much trouble with their breathing from severe COPD . . ."

"Wait—what? Severe? No one said anything about me bein' severe," Dale broke in.

"You must've had some idea your COPD was severe. You can't work, and it limits what you can do. That shouldn't be any surprise."

"I thought everybody who smoked like I did felt this way. So, am I special?"

"Yes, you are specially sick. It *is* severe. It can't get better, though it can be controlled. I think you basically told me that much earlier, Dale, when you said you hadn't been to the hospital emergency since Dr Dryden and the palliative care team stepped in to help you." Dr. Lea paused, but Dale didn't respond.

"As I was saying, most people by this point in time with severe COPD and on the max of their medications and using oxygen have tried another type of medicine I don't see on your record, and Dr. Dryden didn't mention it in his last two visits. It's a type of strong pain medicine; sometimes we use the term "opioid" for a med like this. It's been around for a while but can work to help with your feeling of shortness of breath. It . . ."

"I can finish that sentence. It's morphine. Isn't that right? That's what you were going to say."

"Yes, morphine. How did you know? Tell me what you know?"

"Doc Dryden talked to me about it. We almost tried it, but from my history he decided to wait a while."

"Why is that, Dale?"

"Well, I had problems with pain medicines in the past. For my chronic back pain I was on strong pain medicines, not morphine but others. I ended up taking them for the wrong reasons, and it went on for quite a while; I got into trouble about it and haven't been on them since. I feel my breathing's been helped without them, and I want it to stay that way.

"If you knew me from before, you'd be shocked to be hearing that from my mouth, but it's the truth. I don't want them unless I have to have them, and right now I don't need them."

"Dale, it sure sounds like you and Dr. Dryden worked through these issues together."

"We did. We went back and forth about them—I'd say for over three months or six months, something like that. He was the first doc to be honest—took the time to listen to me and helped me work it out."

He paused before continuing, "And I get the feeling you'd be the same way with me. I wasn't going to talk about it with you today. Even if it was going to be brought up, I wasn't going there. But you seem to be of the same style as Dr. Dryden; you listen, and I get a sense you care. I'm not just another drug history person to you. I trust that if or when you think it's necessary we'll deal with it then. Fair?"

"Fair," Dr. Lea agreed.

"What else do you want to go over today, doc?"

"Yes, well, there is another important topic. It's a document called by different names but usually either advance directive or power of attorney for health care. This isn't a living will or your testamentary will or your funeral plans. I don't see one in your records. Do you have one?"

"No, I don't, but I have a file with several copies of blank papers over there." Dale stepped over the oxygen tubing and walked a few steps to a small table covered with a large pile of papers, loose and sticking out in different directions. He leaned onto the table and paused for a minute. "This is my file cabinet. Can you tell?" His words came out sounding forceful and weak, with a tight, hoarse quality that didn't go unnoticed.

"I guess it works as well as a real one. You knew exactly where they were." Dr. Lea glanced through the pile of papers with one eye watching Dale recover from his breathlessness. "Do you want to talk about this today?"

"Not really. Doc Dryden tried many times, and your social worker, Robert, tried too. Oh, and your nurse did. No one got too far about it. Do you think you can?" Dale challenged while shrugging, grinning and cackling.

"I for sure want to," Dr. Lea stated with zeal. "How about I give you an assignment for next time?" He nodded. "What if you give me five reasons you don't have one completed or why you won't talk about it, and I'll give you five reasons you should have one. Deal?"

"Deal. Hey, I like you. Doc did all right turning me over to you, I can tell already. I'm a good judge of character."

"Before I leave I want to examine you, especially since this is the first time we've met, and I want to have a baseline on your exam findings for me to keep track. Is that okay?"

"Yes, of course. You're the doc." He set the same unlit cigarette, now a little more crumpled from having been held for so long, on the edge of the ashtray by his lamp and chair.

Dr. Lea performed her initial exam, which was more extensive than a follow up visit exam might be. She noted all the usual signs of advanced lung disease; this was a classic case in which all of the physical features lined up to support the diagnosis.

"You're all finished up now, doc? Any surprises?" Dale asked.

"Yes, finished, and no, surprises. Just as I expected. Thanks."

"Well, I see with your packing up your tools, you're done with me." Before he continued Dale waited for her to finish putting away her examination tools and shut down the tablet. "I remember my assignment, and you remember yours. K?"

"Got it, Dale," Dr. Lea replied. "I'll be back in six weeks."

"Sounds good." He held the door for her. "Not feeling too steady right now, so I'll let you go out on your own—careful on those steps. I've been meaning to fix 'em. Careful."

"No problem, Dale. Bye."

8

DALE

PALLIATIVE CARE SUMMARY – 3

Pain Medicine Issues

DALE'S experience with addiction, its related issues, and pain is very common. In fact, many people don't handle these issues as well as he did. However, in light of his prior experience with pain medicine, which he volunteered to Dr. Lea, the reader may have questions regarding pain medication misuse and palliative care. I will review the information about addiction in the introductory material about chronic pain.

This topic is so broad that any discussion here would be incomplete. The points important to palliative care, especially for those dealing with chronic pain, however, are significant. It's essential for the patient to seek the latest specialized care for chronic pain while also getting support from their primary care provider. A thorough approach from a specialist is important, but successful management requires patients to, first and foremost, actively and intentionally address these issues to overcome the negative effects of chronic pain on their lives. Managing it can be complicated and challenging, but having a fully collaborative relationship with one's doctors is crucial.

The process starts with the patient making the right choices and seeking wholeness. This approach definitely includes physical aspects, but the rest of the person also needs to be addressed honestly and completely, including their psychological, social, and spiritual sides.

Let's start by looking at information about addiction.

Addiction

A strong misconception is that the use of strong opioids will always lead to addiction, although it is true that all opioids, along with other controlled medications, carry the risk of causing addiction.

Some people worry about becoming addicted to opioids when they use them for a painful medical condition. This event is rare, especially when the palliative care team closely monitors and manages use. One way of thinking about this is that, when patients feel a lot of pain, the pain medicine can help. On the other hand, when there isn't much pain, having that medication in the body may allow it to be do other, unnecessary things to or within the body instead.

It's important here to explain several key terms* and ideas to assist in better understanding. The patient and those

---

*As a medical professional I use specific resources for medical professionals. For example, with regard to this information I used the American Society of Addiction Medicine (ASAM) to verify my definitions. For the reader as a layperson, I recommend using reputable qualified online websites for your information; they will have similar information directed to you. I am reluctant to provide specific sites by name in order to avoid any conflicts due to what might be considered a recommendation. Search the internet carefully and avoid blogs or sites that only list complaints, as they frequently distort the truth or fail to offer a clear and full picture. You can always contact your medical professional for their opinion and input to specifically address your particular circumstances. These terms can also be applied to other medications besides opioids. They are applicable to any mediations that are habit forming or potentially addictive.

involved with their care need complete information about this topic with the intention of not in any way discouraging the appropriate use of opioid medications:

Addiction: a condition or disease for which a person seeks strong pain medication even though they don't have a significant or serious painful condition. This means that there is no real medical reason for them to have it. They might also engage in unusual or illegal activities to obtain the medicine, despite the fact that there are harmful or negative consequences from it. This person is out of control and acting compulsively.

Tolerance: Tolerance is a normal physiologic response of the body from long-term use of substances such as pain medicine. This effect does not indicate that someone is addicted but is the body's natural reaction to regularly having the medicine in it; the body makes internal adjustments since it is "getting used to" the presence of the medication. When the individual is regularly using pain medicine, the body begins to block receptors that sense pain. However, this can lead to an increase in the number of pain receptors, meaning that the person will need more pain medicine to block those extra receptors. Additionally, as the receptors might become more sensitive to pain, more pain medicine will be needed to reduce its effects.

Strong pain medicine doesn't act directly at the pain location. Instead, it affects the pathway that sends pain signals from the source of the pain to the brain. This usually happens at the transfer points near the spinal cord and in the brain—the points at which the receptors are located—to allow the medicine to take effect. A pain-relieving local anesthetic delivered by injection works differently; it stops pain at the source by blocking the nerves that send pain signals.

It's normal for tolerance to develop, and it is not an indication of addiction. Another reason to have an expert treat someone's pain resulting from a serious illness, such as cancer, is to understand when tolerance is occurring (the patient is feeling more pain with the same amount of pain medicine in their body) or if their condition is worsening and causing more pain. In both situations doctors may consider changing the dosage, as well as possibly adding or adjusting other medications (adjuvant medications) that help the pain medicine work better. This can help treat the pain without the patient needing strong pain medicine, thus lowering the side effects and other long-term effects of opioids.

Pseudo-tolerance: This term refers to the need for a higher amount of medicine to gain relief from symptoms. This might seem like tolerance, but it could actually be caused by the disease progressing and leading to more pain. This was mentioned above under tolerance, but it's an important point.

Withdrawal happens when the body reacts to taking less of a medicine or stopping it altogether. This also happens with other types of medicine. Examples include different types of antidepressants, anti-anxiety medications, antipsychotics, or steroids that are used for a longer period of time. Once the body has gotten used to the medicine (tolerance), stopping it can cause the receptors to overreact and lead to symptoms of withdrawal. These symptoms can vary from mild to severe and can sometimes be fatal. That's why the patient should follow their doctor's prescribing instructions and not change the dosages on their own. A pharmacist can help explain the prescription instructions and withdrawal effects of medications.

Withdrawal symptoms are usually uncomfortable and can vary in seriousness. They often leave the patient feeling opposite the way the medicine affects that receptor.

With withdrawal from pain medicine, the individual may suddenly feel a lot more pain when the medicine stops blocking the pain signals. Receptor blocking can also happen in the gut. When the opioid blocks the receptors it can cause constipation, nausea, or vomiting. When the receptors are suddenly no longer blocked the effect can be diarrhea, stomach cramps, nausea, and vomiting. When other receptors become unblocked and more active during withdrawal, this causes the pupils in the eyes to dilate; increases tears and saliva; and results in sweating, flushed skin, and goosebumps. More serious reactions that affect the brain include lower alertness, signs of coma, severe confusion and agitation, anxiety, and tremors or shaking movements.

It is important for the patient to tell their doctor about these symptoms or go to the emergency room for severe reactions. This way they can receive the right treatment to allow them to feel better and prevent their condition and withdrawal symptoms from getting worse.

Dependence: When the body has reached the point at which it will manifest withdrawal symptoms, this means that it has developed dependence on the medicine. In a sense the body has begun to rely on the medicine being present. It feels more natural to the body to have it present than to function without it. Another way to state this is that, in order for the body to feel right or normal, it wants to have the medicine in its system. Again, this is different from addiction, which is the behavior of going out and seeking drugs in quest of a feeling that often has nothing to do with the normal use of the medicine. Dependence is not addiction but is rather the sign of a normal physiologic response of the body to having the medicine in the system for a period of time. This time frame varies by both the medication and the individual.

Opioid use disorder: OUD occurs when people have progressed to the point of using pain medicine for reasons other than legitimate medical treatment for pain, anxiety, etc. This might be from habit or for self-treatment of anxiety or depression, or the person may be in a quest for social acceptance or for euphoria, the feeling of an opioid high. As a result they struggle to maintain control in terms of proper use of the medicine. The pain might have started from a real medical issue, but now the pain is gone or not serious enough to require strong medicine. Still, the person wants to keep taking it for those other illicit reasons.

This disorder falls under the broader category of substance use disorder. The best way to treat patients with serious illness-related pain, such as pain from cancer, as well as opioid use disorder, is by close collaboration with an expert in addiction medicine and a palliative care specialist. If there is no cooperation between the patient and their medical providers in reducing the use of harmful substances during treatment, the focus must shift to a method called harm reduction therapy, which is part of the addiction specialists' expertise and their team's work. Close and open communication is critical among all the specialists involved.

Overdose and Naloxone: Overdose refers to either the intentional or accidental taking of too much medication at one time. An intentional overdose can be a way of trying to commit suicide or misusing medicine for reasons different from its intended use. If the individual is having thoughts of suicide, there are online resources available, and their doctor can help. If the person is in crisis or needs immediate help, it is best to call an ambulance or go to the emergency room. Reach out to someone for help. Accidental overdose, on the other hand, is just what it says: not an intentional action but resulting from regular use of the medication or unintentional repeat self-dosing, leading to high blood levels and the overdose effects of the medication.

Naloxone is a prescription medication, but in many states or communities it can be obtained without a prescription from a pharmacy—essentially, over-the-counter (OTC). It is used quickly to treat an overdose from strong pain medications. Those strong medications could either be legally obtained with a prescription or could be illegal drugs.

Naloxone doesn't work for other kinds of medicines, such as those used for anxiety or depression. The individual should talk to their doctor or pharmacist for information about their medication and prescription education. It is also wise to check with them once per year about the patient's need for Naloxone. These professionals can provide exact instructions for how to use Naloxone. It's important to know the instructions before the medication is needed, because that situation will be an emergency and might be frightening. A new product is a nasal spray administering a set dose. Please be informed and ready. Naloxone saves lives.

Chronic pain: This is a syndrome with complex definitions, causes, and treatment. It can begin with a sudden pain or injury but is a completely different condition from the pain I talk about in this book. To properly and successfully recognize, diagnose, and treat chronic pain, the doctor and team need special skills, training, and certification.

It is best to address chronic pain in a clinic where different medical experts work together with the doctor to perform a thorough evaluation and comprehensive treatment plan. This takes time. The team will include a pain doctor, a nurse, a psychologist, a social worker, a pharmacist, a physical therapist, an occupational therapist, and other professionals. Treatment involves using medicine and at times procedures (sometimes called interventions) designed to reduce pain. They will also include the patient's primary care doctor, since they know the patient best.

Opioid contracts and trust: Opioid contracts are now nearly universal when a patient and physician or prescriber together decide it is time to use strong pain medicine. Some states require a legal document to be discussed and signed before the doctor can prescribe pain medicine to the patient. This may seem like a lot to ask, but it is important for both the doctor and the patient to make sure the patient understands how to use these medicines correctly and safely. The physician will usually explain what counts as improper use that can cause the prescription to be stopped. Be careful with these medications; this is serious.

———

Pain and chronic pain, as I have indicated, are not the same. Most of the pain treated by palliative care professionals is cancer related: pain in the body caused by cancer. The palliative care team can help with different types of serious pain from illnesses, depending on the type of pain, its pattern, the treatment being used, and what is causing it. The physician and patient will decide this together after fully understanding the situation. This includes an appropriate evaluation, a review of medical records, and possibly getting help from other specialists to better understand the complex condition and symptoms.

Additional information and observations about chronic pain are included in other sections of this book, as applicable. But more thorough content is available in the Appendix. Recognize again that management of chronic pain is a specialty for which the patient's primary care provider may have extra training and experience to assist them. They are the patient's first contact for obtaining information and finding the right help. Online self-help has its limits; the patient needs a full team to manage chronic pain successfully.

9

PEARL

PATRICK'S STORY

Ten Years Earlier

PEARL didn't know what to do. She was holding her head in her hands, looking down at the floor and feeling her body rocking to the steady beeps of Patrick's heartbeat on the ICU monitor. Patrick was lying in the hospital bed, unresponsive. *He would know what to do, but he can't tell me. Why didn't we talk about this? We talked about everything else in the world, but certainly not about stuff as important as this is. We talked about the bills and the checkbook balance, the kids, the grandkids. We talked about Christmas and the gifts this year for everyone. Why not give me this gift? This final gift? It would be the best Christmas gift ever. We talked about cars breaking down. The furnace needing a checkup. We talked about the World Series and the Super Bowl. But why didn't we talk about what to do if this happened to either one of us!*

Pearl kept this up for a while; she didn't keep track of how many times the hospital nurse or other staff came and went in Patrick's hospital room. She knew she had sat like this for a while, as her back was noticeably aching, and it hadn't been upon their arrival. Patrick has been in the ICU now for five days. It seemed like five years in her mind and heart.

With no chance of surviving this massive, bleeding stroke involving the cerebrum and the brainstem, where the body's automatic system controls are located, Patrick would not be long for this world.

Five days they gave him to recover before making decisions—for me to make the decisions. Without Patrick helping me. Either I have to decide to make his body live longer with an artificial surgical feeding tube and a permanent breathing tube that will allow to him live indefinitely until his body quit from something else—I can't remember what they said it would be—or I have to decide to stop the aggressive care and allow him to die naturally from the results of this stroke. They told me that when he dies it won't be from "pulling the plug" but from the critical stroke damage his brain can never recover from.

That was supposed to keep me from feeling any kind of guilt about his dying after taking away the life support. It does help, but I have to keep convincing myself every few minutes. Erin and Patrick Jr. are no help; they keep saying it's up to me, that they'll support me in whatever I decide—Thanks!

Lord, we haven't talked in a while. You know what's going on here. Help me to know and decide what to do. What is best for Patrick?

Pearl had feared this decision day would come since the moment she found out what was wrong with Patrick. She'd had the sense from the start that he wasn't going to recover. She saw how he looked before the ambulance came to pick him up. She knew. But that didn't help with the decision-making. If only Patrick had given a clue of what he would have wanted in this situation.

Pearl looked over at him while holding his hand. The hand that had been so big and strong when they'd first met; her hand could have disappeared in it if he'd held it just right. She smiled and teared up, remembering their first handhold while they'd walked from a downtown festival event. His hand now was fragile looking; the skin appeared pale . . . frail . . . thin. . . and pearlescent, almost lifeless in her hand now.

How did we get to this point and not realize it? I can't make him linger like this. I know what he'd want—or wouldn't want. He wouldn't want to exist in this shell of a body, without any chance of recovery. There's no way he would want that. He'd feel like we're trapping his soul—who he really is—in a body instead of letting him truly live, more whole than he is here on earth. I guess I could think of releasing him as him getting healed. He does have faith and hope, and that's supposed to give me peace since I know he'll be in heaven; I have that faith too. Lord, I know you're with me. I know what I have to do. Let him go to his final rest—it's his time. Patrick, I give you back to the Lord.

Oh, and Lord, let me not put my family through this turmoil.

10

PEARL

STABLE SYMPTOMS, MORE TO SAY

Two Months After Last Visit

"PEARL," Dr. Lea began, "It's been seven months since we started caring for you here at the palliative care clinic. Let's summarize where we've been. Is that okay with you?"

"Yes, that's fine. Do you want me to start?"

"Sure. What has been the most important part of those months to you?"

"Well first, having a team led by you that's focused on my symptoms and not distracted by all the rest of what's going on with me. That makes a big difference. Your team—they genuinely want to know how I'm doing and figure out how to help me in the best way possible. They seem to sincerely care about me. You just don't see that very often in this day and age. It gives me peace of mind and confidence. That's the most important thing.

"The second thing is like the first; you and the PC team (that's what I call them), want to know how my symptoms are and make a plan to help them. You really understand my pain related to my disease and know the medications in fine detail—unlike any other doctors and nurses I've had. You're truly experts! That I can say without a doubt. I can shout it from the mountaintops if you'd like!"

"No, no, that's okay. You've said enough, Pearl. We're glad to hear you're satisfied and pleased and that our efforts are improving your life in a real and lasting manner. Tell me more about how much it has helped in terms of what you can do on a day-to-day basis. Or some of the things you can do now that you couldn't before."

"Well, my fatigue is the biggest trouble, and though I've resisted any of your or your team's suggestions, I know you're looking out for my best interests—and when I'm ready I know you'll be willing to help me." *I see Dr. Lea nodding, and with her eye contact I know she's listening and is in this for me.* "Even though I haven't used any of your suggestions, you aren't frustrated with me—or at least I can't tell you are." Pearl winked and smiled.

"You've allowed me the choice of continuing the Tykitrol treatment for the leukemia, and that gives me the hope of the medicine keeping the disease from worsening more quickly. I know from what you've said that 'there's no proof' it will work, but it still gives me a feeling of control. The tradeoff of fatigue for this continued hope helps me accept what's going on with me. For now I still want it—to save you the question, doctor." Pearl paused, looking down.

Dr. Lea preserved the silence. *I don't want to interrupt Pearl's train of thought here. I think she's getting ready to tell me something more.*

"With the pain—it hasn't been the worst of my symptoms, but I know you and your team are very concentrated on it." *Again, Dr. Lea's nodding helps me to know she and her team are for me wholeheartedly.* "I appreciate that you didn't come in and change my medications all around, that you worked with what had been effective and then modified it last time from a small change in my pain. I trust you that—if my pain gets worse, as I fear . . . and especially with your focus on it, I more than likely expect it to—I trust your decision on pain medication changes." Pearl again paused, and another silence ensued.

"This may not sound like a big deal to you, considering what you do all day long as a doctor, but to me it was a big deal. So, thank you." This time Pearl stopped and reached into her purse. *Oh, rats. I didn't want to cry. But it means so much to me. I wish Patrick had had this kind of attention; he needed and deserved it. We didn't know about the possibility then, and no one told us.* Pearl dabbed her eyes lightly in the corners and then continued, holding the tissue clutched in her hand.

"I've got to mention the whole ordeal with the power of attorney thing," Pearl went on. "I'm sorry—you call it advance directive." *Another knowing nod.* "That was worth it, though. Maybe just as important as the fatigue and pain I mentioned. I have peace about it. I'm glad for the changes I made, as hard as they were. And the encouragement to do it and the suggestions of how to do it you and Robert and the nurse gave me helped so much. My son was troubled—upset, really—but only for a short time that day we talked. He eventually saw my point and agreed his sister was the best one to handle the medical decisions for me. He continues to be first on the financial decisions.

"So, for all that, Dr. Lea, I'm grateful and glad your team is on my side." *There, I made it through.*

"Thanks, Pearl. I understand. It can be tough going through those conversations, but in the end it's for the best. I'm so glad you've followed through. Just remember to share it with your doctors and hospital."

"I have already."

"Your pain—how did the medication change work for you?"

"It helped, and I continue with it the same way."

"Pearl, tell me about some of the things you can do."

"I would say I'm not doing anything now that I wasn't before, but I can continue to do what's important to me. Keeping up on my place. I can still go to the store and the hairdresser. I go and visit with my friends. I can see my family. These are not extraordinary things but ones I value and want to keep up with. Very important to me. I think you can tell."

Pearl knew the routine of climbing onto the exam table at the end of the doctor's questions for the exam. So far the results were always the same, but Dr. Lea performed the exam anyway. No changes.

Dr. Lea stepped back from the exam table. "Pearl, tell me about your name. For all your Irish background, I know Pearl isn't an Irish name—I looked it up. Do you know the story there?"

"Yes, I do. You're right, and it is an interesting story. Both my mother and father are Irish. I married Patrick—he was mostly Irish too. The story goes that my mother loved pearls and wanted to name a daughter the Irish name for pearls. But it's a very old name and awkward here in the US. It's Máiréad, pronounced Mah-Rade, derived from Margaret. So, even though she preferred the older Irish name, she named me Pearl. Once in a while she did call me Máiréad; she liked that. That's why my daughter's name is Eireann, which is the Irish traditional spelling for Erin."

"That's interesting. I have a similar story for my first name, Lea. My mom really preferred the more traditional Irish girl's name spelled with the accents over the e and a, but she figured that would have caused lots of confusion, and she spared me some embarrassment too."

Pearl smiled. "I wondered about that."

"Having it spelled that way would have been traditional, but as it is it's not spelled how it sounds in Irish," Dr. Lea noted.

"Yes, the correct way to pronounce would have been Lay-ah. Correct?"

"Yes, that's right. My mother was from Hebrew ancestry but married an Irishman. She wanted to name me Leah, the Hebrew name with the *h* on the end, but, keeping with the Irish tradition on my father's side, she chose to use the spelling closer to the traditional Irish version. Our stories are very similar." *Interesting.* "Thanks for sharing. I've always preferred people to call me Dr. Lea and not Dr. Glendale. What about your son's name?"

"His is easy—Patrick. Just like his father's."

"Pearl, I think we've settled all we can today. How about we meet again in three months? You have good symptom control. We're not making any changes. We have a copy of your updated advance directive in our record for you. Does that sound all right—three months?"

"Yes, Dr. Lea. I'll set that up on my way out today. Thank you."

Hugs this time.

11

PEARL

FUNNY DAYS

Three Weeks Later

DR. Lea took a deep, satisfying breath as she walked through the medical staff entrance to Community General Hospital. This time she was there as an attending physician on the medical staff of the hospital that had been home to her post-graduate (after medical school) education for eight years. She knew the hospital's every corner and shortcut through the stairwells to get quickly between floors, as well as the turns to the long hallways over to the outpatient tower and medical education office.

This wasn't her first time back at the hospital since she'd graduated from her palliative care fellowship, but those had been trips down the escalator from the lobby to the educational suite of conference rooms. For those sessions she hadn't arrived through the medical staff entrance but through the public front entrance in the lobby and then down the escalator to her left.

This time she felt some freedom from the burden of house staff working hours; on-call duties with nights, weekends, and holidays; and the endless bustle. She stopped and reflected on this for a moment, enjoying another deep breath. Her new attending physician badge worked fine; there were no mishaps when she signed in at the console by the entrance.

To be honest with herself, she missed the intensity of the hospital and the very sick patients she had cared for over the years, but she didn't miss the frequent calls and the nights of being on call in the ICU. Those she had dreaded, except when there had been a particularly critical patient. At such times her adrenaline rush had kept her keenly aware and focused, and she felt she had learned best at those times.

She had been forced to learn quickly on those occasions, having had to consider simultaneously the patient's clinical situation and the necessary medical literature reading or studying. The learning in those circumstances had also stuck with her. Her feeling at such times was that the knowledge helped not only her but also her patients. Then there was nothing comparable to the incredible satisfaction of getting the patient through their critical illness.

During her last year in the palliative care fellowship after her critical care training years, she'd had to eventually admit to herself that she was enjoying the same degree of satisfaction and sometimes even more. Switching from critical care (a move that hadn't been popular with her attending intensivists, who had expected her to join their hospital group coverage) to palliative care right away had made the most sense in light of what she had witnessed happening in the critical care unit day after day, night after night, patient after patient.

"Hi, Lea, are you back for more? Are you thinking about returning to the hospital? We'll always have a place for you!" It was Troy Needmore, the lead intensivist in the critical care unit and director of the intensivist training program. He was briskly walking in his usual manner, with the tapping sounds of his patent leather shoes echoing through the hallway, the European leather pouch crossing his chest bobbing rhythmically with each step.

He stopped abruptly to talk to her, nearly spilling his tall coffee—and she unintentionally stiffened her spine. She was recalling the emergency pericardiocentesis she had performed with him that still made her start to sweat and her pulse to rush. She had performed the procedure nearly flawlessly . . . except for the single drop of blood that had landed on Dr. Needmore's brand new patent leather shoe. She had never forgotten it—and neither had he. *Why didn't he wear protective shoe covers that day? Or clinical clogs like every other attending did in the ICU? Or something besides brand new patent . . . leather . . . shoes?*

"No, nothing like that." She smiled, having missed his energy and expertise, but not his intensity and demands. She had often thought over the years how he had matched his career choice perfectly with his name. Like other situations with a dentist named Pain or a urologist named Stone. She hurried on, trying to settle her heart rate and concerned that he might speed off without warning before she could finish what she had to say:

"I'm more than happy with my palliative care outpatient clinic and the house calls I do—much different from my years here but equally satisfying. Miss all of you, of course. I like making a difference for people in this way. Every day I use what I learned from you and the hospital staff here at CGH, for which I'm hugely grateful. I know where to go if I ever have the urge to return, and I'll let you know first. But I don't see that happening, thank you."

"Oh, Lea, you never know. The door is always open. Gotta run. Oh, wait. What are you doing here then?"

"The hospital's palliative care team is seeing her to manage her palliative needs while an inpatient; I wanted to see her to see how she is doing."

"Well, come along with me—I'm heading there now too. I promise not to quiz you on the intricacies of metabolic acidosis and EKG changes or on thyrotoxic storms or your favorite, as I recall, of hyponatremia work up. I promise."

Unlikely, was her thought as she quickly fell into step with his cadence to the elevator banks for the ride up to the seventh floor ICU. She didn't listen to the rest of his chitchat about his latest Maserati purchase and French Riviera trip. But she was recalling all too clearly the havoc he had caused her in not allowing her a hybrid position in both critical care and palliative care.

He had stated unequivocally that there would be conflicts of interest in his unit with a dual role like that—which had been the real reason she couldn't have brought herself to return to working for him. Lea didn't strongly resent him; she just didn't want to live her life that way. She had chosen wisely for herself, she recognized, and she had no regrets.

The elevator door rang as they arrived, and she heard him say goodbye and something like "Don't be a stranger." She waved to him as he walked off toward his office in the opposite direction. She wanted to see the nursing staff and a couple of the other doctors to catch up briefly—and Pearl Murphy.

———

Pearl's room

Dr. Lea entered Pearl's room. There was a visitor with her, sitting in the bedside recliner. She looked to be the age of Pearl's daughter—as it turned out she was. *Pearl looks better than I thought she might.* Dr. Lea based this on her visual inspection, comparing her to other patients she had cared for in the past who had been critically ill from sepsis. Pearl had the usual venous access lines, the oxygen tubing to her nose, and the ubiquitous monitor reflecting her current vital signs, both digital and graphically displayed with color, all within normal limits.

Her eyes were closed, her breathing not labored. And her skin not as pale as the doctor would have expected. Both arms lay straight on top of the sheets. The daughter looked up.

"Pearl, it's Dr. Lea, here to visit you." Dr. Lea looked straight into her face, her eyes awaiting acknowledgment. It came swiftly.

"Dr. Lea, so glad to see you. You found me." Pearl reached up to take her hands, with a weakened squeeze for sure, the doctor noted. "This is my daughter, Eireann. Dr. Lea."

"Pleased to meet you, Erin. I've enjoyed taking care of your mom at the palliative care clinic. Delightful lady."

"Thank you, Dr. Lea. Mom's told me all about you and was hoping you'd come to see her and maybe give your opinion on things," Erin replied. She quickly let go of the doctor's hand.

"Okay, thank you, Erin. I will." *She plopped down rather hard into the chair. Is she okay with how her mom is doing? She should be, based on my quick assessment. I'll look through the record to see if there's anything else ominous going on. Or is there something else happening in the family? Or maybe she's just tired . . . ?*

"I'm going to look through your chart on the computer right here." Pearl nodded and closed her eyes, and Erin leaned back, rearranged a blanket, and poked at her phone.

Dr. Lea discovered how sick Pearl had really been when she had arrived at the CGH four days earlier. The patient had been in septic shock and unresponsive, with early acute renal failure, electrolyte disturbance, low hemoglobin, an elevated white cell count, positive blood and urine cultures, and a possible lower GI bleed; these were all listed in her active problem list and diagnoses. She had since received aggressive medical treatment with fluids but had been given no blood transfusions, and she had been put on broad-spectrum antibiotics until results of the cultures were known so focused antibiotic therapy could be started. She was not intubated or in respiratory failure.

"Well, Pearl, I've looked through most of your record on this hospitalization, and you are clearly improving, based on your labs and the doctor's progress notes. I'm looking for your advance directive, and as I'm clicking on your documents section right now I can see . . . yes, your document is uploaded in here, and it's the latest version you just had signed and witnessed. Good.

"Pearl, how are you feeling today compared to yesterday or the day before?"

"I don't remember much from a couple days ago, and yesterday seems kind of foggy to me. But today I feel clear minded but tired and generally blah."

"That's about right for what you've gone through. Erin, do you have any questions or concerns? I'm not in charge of her care or of writing any orders on her, but if I can help answer questions or address any concerns you might have, I'd be happy to do that." Dr. Lea stood now at the foot of the bed next to Erin, who still sat in the recliner, though she had set down the phone next to her in the chair. *Maybe I can go a little further with Erin and see how she's handling all this.*

Erin sat looking out the large window toward the city skyline. It was a dreary day outside, though the rain had lifted, and low hanging clouds were rising upward; however, the lit-up hospital room was bright enough to reflect Erin's expression in the large window.

"Did I wait too long to bring her in?" she asked.

"No, not at all!"

"Mom—she was so . . . funny."

"What do you mean?"

"She was hilarious with her comments and things she was saying about other family members. Making fun of them, in a way. I mean the things she was saying. Stuff like I had left her at a party at someone's home I didn't know, and she wanted me to take her out for bangers and mash—she knows you can't get that around here, not that she'd be into it anyway. She didn't know my name and was beginning to accuse me of meeting up with her husband, Patrick. That's my dad, who died several years ago.

"It was getting weirder by the minute. So unlike her! I don't know—I thought 'Is she sick'? She had no fever or vomiting or rash. Or is it her cancer causing this? So, I decided to call her doctor's office, and they told me to take her in right away. It was just that day she acted funny like that."

"Sounds to me like this funny day was what is called medically an acute delirium. You did exactly the right thing at the right time." Erin relaxed a little in her posture.

"What does that mean? Delirium? Is she going crazy? You mean like Alzheimer's?" Erin's eyebrows shot up as she asked it.

Dr. Lea replied calmly and steadily, "Yes and no. Delirium has nothing at all to do with dementia or Alzheimer's. It's a temporary episode of confusion, though it can be severe and lead to worsening of the sudden acute condition. Sometimes they can get combative and . . . if it's not recognized promptly or treated properly, it can be fatal. It's usually caused by something medical going on suddenly in the body. It can be caused by medicine, disease, or what is sometimes called a metabolic disturbance.

"Lab results can show it most of the time, and that's the case with your mom. There are many possibilities, and she had several conditions based on her presentation to the hospital at the emergency department. They began treating her for it in the emergency room right away; that's what helped her so much.

"Erin, has she had spells like this before?"

"Umm, maybe. I recall something like it but much milder. And she had it for a few more days. She ended up having a bladder infection, I think," Erin recalled.

"That's right," Pearl seconded. 'It was about a year or so ago. I didn't have to come to the hospital. But it was a bladder infection." Her eyes remained closed. "I remember that time much better than I do this one."

"You're tracking with us, Pearl. That's good," Dr. Lea asserted.

"Of course," Pearl stated with emphasis, this time with open eyes.

"Do either of you have any questions or other concerns?"

Both Pearl and Erin shook their heads.

"Okay. Pearl, how is your usual kind of pain? Have they been giving you your regular pain medicine?"

"I can't recall if they have or not. Can you tell from the chart?" Pearl asked.

"Yes, let me check in the record again. Let me see . . ." Dr. Lea's voice trailed off as she navigated through the chart.

"Yes, I see it now. They're giving it to you as we have it planned. And there's a notation saying they had contacted the PC clinic staff for the dosing. Well, good." This was a fine example of good communication between the inpatient and outpatient services. So many times when that doesn't happen the pain gets out of control, and the patient suffers for it.

"Good. Well, you're all set. Before you leave the hospital, they'll set up—or should I say move up?—your appointment to see me within a week after you're discharged. This will be instead of the three-month appointment we already have on the schedule. Okay?"

"If I remember," Pearl stated somewhat vaguely.

"Oh, they'll take care of it for you before you leave. Good to see you improving. You'll probably leave the ICU soon—I mean in the next couple days, probably."

"Thanks for stopping by," Pearl said. "Say, you really seem to know your way around this place."

"I should, I trained here for nearly eight years. So I've been around the block a time or two. I even ran into my old chief trainer on my way in."

"Thanks for seeing Mom today, and for talking to me about my concerns," Erin offered. "That really helped me out. I feel much better about things." Erin shook Dr. Lea's hand but didn't drop it so quickly this time.

"Goodbye. I'll see you at your next appointment, Pearl." With that Dr. Lea turned and left the room.

"I see why you like her," Erin commented to her mom. But Pearl didn't hear her. Her eyes were closed, and the blankets were slowly rising and falling with her slow, steady breathing. Erin smiled and relaxed back into the chair.

12

DALE

UNEXPECTED TALENT CONTEST

Six Weeks Later

DR. Lea stepped into the living room. *I don't believe in déjà vu, but this must be what it's like. Nothing is changed in the house, absolutely nothing! It's just as I left it. Did he even move from his chair? I hope we can make some progress today.*

Dr. Lea shook Dale's hand after she had tried to start an elbow bump greeting, but Dale was having none of that. His big right hand stretched out to shake hers.

"Doc, welcome back," Dale greeted. "You're here for some more with me?"

"Yes, I'm anxious to see how you're doing?"

"You mean how I'm feeling or how I did with my assignment?"

"Both."

"You start," he invited.

"Okay, we'll start with your symptoms, then I'll check you over, and then we'll talk about your assignment."

"Okay, Doc. You're saving the best for last. I did your assignment up big, but you'll have to wait now."

"All right," Dr. Lea agreed, drawing her words out slowly with the almost questioning tone of someone trying to figure something out while talking. *So, what is Dale up to this time?* She retrieved her stethoscope at the same time, smiling to herself.

Dr. Lea finished her examination efficiently, noting that his exam findings were the same as on her first visit. She mostly noticed how diminished his breath sounds were, with what seemed to be very little airflow back and forth with the deep, deliberate breaths she asked him to take. His heart sounds were distant and regular, as expected. He had the nail clubbing indicative of low oxygen associated with advanced COPD and the chronic respiratory failure that came with it. Dale's fingernails were also discolored from his nicotine habit. At *least they aren't cyanotic*, she thought. His mild edema of the lower legs was unchanged, and his vital signs were stable.

"Well, your exam is the same as last time, Dale."

"That's good, right, doc?"

"Yes and no. Yes, it's good in that it doesn't show any changes from before, but no in the sense that it does continue to show the advanced lung disease, as expected."

"Got it, doc."

After jotting notes from the exam, Dr. Lea continued, "Dale, tell me how you're breathing feels. How would you rate your feeling of shortness of breath?"

"The breathing is the same as always. I'm taking all my meds and neb'lizers and oxygen. Yes, I'm careful with the smoking. I turn the oxygen off. I'm not interested in blowing up myself or the place. Rate it? I'd say medium to bad."

"Can you give it a number? Your medium and bad might be different from what I think that feels like."

"Seven, then. Maybe seven and a half . . . No, just kidding, a seven."

The rest of the review of his symptoms went the same way. Dale denied or downplayed his symptoms as the doctor questioned him.

"Okay, I want to hear your five best reasons for why you don't want to fill out the advance directive forms."

"Okay, I'll be right back." Dale left the living room and disappeared down the hallway. "Hannah!" Dale called out. She left the kitchen without saying anything and followed him down the hallway. Their voices were muffled from the distance, and there was the competing noise of the oxygen concentrator running. The two appeared to be behind a door partway down the hallway. There was the sound of a box falling from the same direction.

"Everything okay?" Dr. Lea called out. There was no answer, so she made her way down the hallway too. When she was partway there, she was startled to hear a guitar being strummed. Dr. Lea moved back to the living room and sat down. *What is going on?*

Several minutes later Dale and Hannah appeared from down the hallway. He was carrying a guitar, and Hannah was keeping track of the oxygen tubing to prevent a fall.

"Well, doc. Six weeks gave me plenty of time to come up with five reasons, so I decided to write a little song I put to music for you. It's not polished up, but I'm proud of it." Dale's grin was wide.

"I'm surprised! I had no idea you played a guitar or even wrote music."

"Well, we'll see if you call it music or not."

"I'm sure it will be good."

"Here it goes." And Dale began strumming, pausing to announce, "I call it 'The First Is the Worst.'"

"The new doc gave it to me,
An assignment to complete.
I gave it some thought
And this came to me.

I don't like talking about it
Because it makes me feel afraid.
What's going to happen
To me, to me. I'm afraid.

So that's reason one
And I've got four more to go.
But to me the first
Is undeniably the worst.

Yes, the first is the worst.

Here's number two
For me to tell you.
I don't know where to start
Someone will have to help me,
I can't understand it
No less afford it, it, it
From the at-tor-ney.

Yes, the first is the worst.

After two comes three,
It is much like two
Or is it one?
I don't want to make it happ'n
If I just men-shun.

Yes, the first is the worst.

Now comes number four
I'm almost done,
Can you believe that, Hon?
Oh, wait, Hon . . . she's not here,
Oh, my . . . oh my dear.
What if they "yank the plug,"
Too soon, way, way too soon?
What ever am I to do?

Yes, the first is the worst.

On to number five,
and then I'm done.
I don't mean that way
Cause I want to live.
I'm not that bad off, am I doc?
Tell me the truth . . . I think, doc
You know what to do,
Just do what you think is best,
For me, that is, not for the rest.
I don't want you or anyone else
To give up on me yet.

Yes, the first is the worst.

But now I'm done,
And it's all complete.
I made it, I made it a Repeat.
But then am I curst?
Yes, the first is the worst."

"What do you think, doc? How'd I do on my assignment?"
Dale looked at Dr. Lea, who was blank faced. "Doc, did you

get it?" He let the guitar slump onto his lap, his hope turning to quickly to despair.

"I've never, ever, had anyone sing their reasons *against*, let alone *for* completing their advance directive. Never. Oh, I got it, all right.

"You shocked me! I didn't know you were so musically talented. It was beautiful. It really was. I . . . I can't get over it. Did you play with a group or record something before? It sounds so professional. I'm sorry, but I was totally not expecting that.

"I mean, I thought you might even forget to do it or just plain refuse. That's what I thought. I'm sorry. I judged you all wrong. It's beautiful."

"Thanks, doc. Don't get all teary eyed with me, now. I don't have any tissues around. You'll have to use your own sleeve."

"Oh, you're fine. Dale, tell me more about your music career. Sounds like more than a flash in the pan."

"Well, doc, not a whole lot to tell. It was over in a hurry. The short story is through a few music connections from a lot of coincidences that fell into place, I made it to Nashville. And worked as a studio acoustic guitar player. I like to write songs and strum the guitar. One of mine got noticed by a lead singer, Billy Ray Thomas . . ."

"Hey, I've heard of him!" Dr. Lea exclaimed.

"Not surprised—he won some awards and such. But one of mine made it as a finalist for the top Billboard Country song of the year; it was called "Cloud Burst Monday." But a tragedy struck the group, and it fell apart—kind of like a country music song, really. I went into hiding, I guess you could call it. But I still like to write songs now and then and play them for myself now that Linda's gone. Nobody else around much except Hannah—she tolerates me—and now Aaron in the last weeks."

"Fascinating story. Unexpected," Dr. Lea added finally. "Now I've got to hold up my end of the deal."

"That's right. Your turn," Dale responded with evident glee. Eagerly he rubbed his hands together in impatient anticipation of the competition.

"I'll try after your overture. Shall I do it in reverse order? Start with reason number five and go backward down to number one?"

"Oh, so you're going Letterman-style on me? It's not totally original but creative, I'll have to say. Go for it. Too bad you couldn't do it like he did with the Top Ten."

"All right, let me see . . . Give me a minute and I'll start with number ten." Dr. Lea jotted some notes for a few minutes that made Dale wonder whether she could follow through, but his liking for a contest made him gloat. He uncharacteristically held back, even leaning back to give her a chance. He waited.

"Doc?"

"Just about ready for you, Dale," she remarked with a wry smile. Dale was still feeling confident, though slightly less so than a few minutes earlier. He picked up his guitar and began to strum out the tune of "The First is the Worst."

"That's not going to distract me, if you're trying." Dr. Lea didn't look up as she wrote more; she was scribbling more quickly and using arrows to indicate the right order for her Top Ten. When she had finished and looked it over, she sat back and tapped her cheek in concentration. Dale kept right on strumming, now humming the melody. Then he began to play the Jeopardy theme song as he waited for her.

"Hey, I hear that," Dr. Lea commented. "Okay, I'm ready. Here it goes. Wait! I need a theme song."

"How about this one?" Dale began. He began to play and started to sing: "A long, long time ago, I can still remember how that music used to make me feel. Wait, it makes me *smile*."

"Okay, that's enough. No more of the Don McLean song."

"Hey, I wanted a chance to sing the line: 'So Bye-bye Miss American Pie.'"

"Too late, I'm ready now. Here it goes:

"The Top Ten reasons for completing an advance directive, Letterman-style:

"Number Ten: It helps your attorney. Maybe a bad joke on this one, but I think Letterman would say it.

"Number Nine: It resolves conflict.

"Number Eight: You get better care.

"Number Seven: It's a conversation starter.

"Number Six: It sets an example.

"Number Five: It gives clear direction.

"Number Four: It gives burden relief.

"Number Three: You are treated the way you want.

"Number Two: You make sure.

"And, drum roll please!" Dale thumped once on the guitar body.

"And Number One: Peace of mind."

Dale nodded in approval. "Not bad, doc. Not bad at all. I'd say it's a tie."

"Good, I agree," Dr. Lea smiled. "And it's easier to explain than the meaning of McLean's 'American Pie.'"

"Whoa, good one, doc." Dale drummed on his guitar while applause was heard from the kitchen, from Hannah.

"I vote for Dr. Lea's performance and break the tie!" Hannah exclaimed.

"Oh, great!" Dale replied with a sarcastic tone, meaning more like, "You would!

"No ganging up on me—it's my home that's hosting this talent show event."

They all laughed.

Dr. Lea began, "Yes, really let me explain, because I think it will help address your concerns from your five points you made in your ballad.

"First of all, I can certainly see you're afraid. You sang about it through your whole song. And I can understand where you're coming from. If I may speak personally now, I didn't want to lose my mom, and not talking about her advanced cancer seemed to help keep it all away. It didn't, of course, but it felt that way. As time went by the reality of the disease continued with its relentless pace and progress. We had to deal with it. And I think for you it's similar.

"You don't have cancer, and the course of your advanced chronic lung disease is far different, but it is going to progress. Everyone's case is different, so hard to predict, and I'm not asking you for permission to make any predictions for you . . . unless you want to talk about that." Dale shook his head no.

Dr. Lea continued, "But you're not anywhere near progressing to the end—you're not what I'd call trending toward hospice. Remember that hospice is different from palliative care. With hospice the condition is terminal, meaning that the person has a prognosis of a life expectancy of six months or less. Your condition is stable; you're weakened and affected by your condition but not nearing the end of your life at this time. So, this is the best time to talk about what kind of care you want and how you want it.

"Just talking about it won't make it happen. And it's best to talk about it before a crisis hits, when someone else will have to figure out what you would prefer in the middle of a medical crisis. That's not good planning."

After a brief pause she resumed talking, noting that he was looking at her but not trying to break into the conversation at that moment.

"We can help you; I mean the palliative care team has experience to help you work through thinking about it, and you can do so without an attorney or spending money on it. There are reasons going to a lawyer can be helpful, but it isn't necessary. The PC team is aware of the laws in our state and knows the requirements to complete the documents so they'll be correct, complete, and legal. That doesn't mean they'll tell you what to do or what to put in them, but they will guide you in their completion.

"Then, when the paperwork is completed, your doctors and the hospital will know exactly what you prefer for your care when a choice becomes necessary. I've said a lot, and you've been listening. Do you have any questions? Or is there something I can clarify for you?"

"No, doc. I've heard most of that before, but you do have a catchy way of explaining it. I don't feel as afraid." He thought for a moment and then rendered his verdict: "Not ready today."

"That's fine, I want you to think it over. I want you to be absolutely convinced this is right before you do it.

"Remember, this is your document explaining your wishes. So that no one will "yank the plug" too soon. as you put it; it will be in your timing (because you'll have set down in your words when to say 'Enough is enough'). We're not going to tell you when that is. If you don't spell it out, then someone else will have to do it based on the way they *think* you would want it. By completing the paperwork you'll be making it easier on the person you choose as your decision-maker—in a way you can consider it your gift to them—your last gift to your family.

"It'll relieve their stress and assure you of the care you want the way you want it. You're in charge. Whether the help involves a ventilator or breathing machine or CPR—you know, chest compressions—or kidney dialysis or feeding tubes if you can't eat any more and you aren't going to recover, your treating team will know clearly what your choices are. That way they can plan and not have to wait for someone else to make up their mind on what to do if there are disagreements in the family. So, it can help resolve or avoid conflicts.

"Lots to think over," Dr. Lea murmured.

"Sure is . . ." Dale stopped. "Are you done?"

"Not quite, but almost. And then, when you're done with that—when the paperwork is completed, signed, witnessed, and then given to the hospital and your doctors—you won't have to do anything else with it. Unless, of course, you want to change it. You can do that anytime, as long as your mind and thinking are still clear. It's good to review the directive once in a while, at least every year or so if there's any big change in your condition.

"Then, finally, when the forms are completed you can go on living, knowing that your wishes are recorded and your decision-maker has been chosen. At that point you can have my number One on the list: peace. Peace in knowing that your wishes are known and will be followed, so you won't have to stress over these issues. Now, *that's* peace, don't you think, Dale?"

"You bet." Dale waited, and the doctor gave him time to think. "My only close relative I'd want to have involved is my son. His name is Aaron. I don't want it to burden anyone else."

"Don't think of it as burden. After your advance direct . . ."

"Look, Doc. I've got a lot going on in my mind. You've given me plenty to think about. Okay? I need some time. Thank you—I mean it, but I've heard enough for now. There's more to my story. Some of it I may not want to tell, and some of it I might. I don't know right now. Okay? Please." Dale motioned with his arm toward the front door.

"Look, Dale, I'm sorry if I overwhelmed you. I thought you were tracking with me and didn't have anything to say, so I kept on going. Sorry for that. I'm not trying to make it more difficult for you—really, I'm not." Dr. Lea reached down to put her equipment away into her bag, and Dale reached over to light a cigarette, not watching her.

Hannah couldn't be seen by either one, but, silent in the kitchen, she held her hands to her face to quiet her mewling.

"Doc, stop," Dale directed suddenly. She waited with her hand on the doorknob before turning toward Dale's voice coming from the recliner. He was puffing out cigarette smoke, but she could see the oxygen tubing he'd thrown across the room.

"Doc, come back in two weeks. That'll be enough time. Can't promise another song in that time, but it'll be enough. Deal?"

"Deal. See you in two weeks, Dale."

13

DALE

A LOT OF "NEVERS" TAKEN CARE OF, AND SOME SURPRISES

Two Weeks Later

"DOC, come on in! What do you notice?" Dale asked.

"Dale, that's obvious. First, there's no blue smoke haze in the air. I know you've kept from smoking during our visits, but this is real change. Congratulations! You quit smoking?"

"I did! Good job, doc. What else?" Dale was nearly giddy as he asked it.

"Well, let me see. There's light in the room." *I notice he trimmed his beard, had a haircut, and has clean clothes on. But I'm not sure I want to eagerly agree right away that I noticed these personal changes. Part of me is suspicious that he's being capricious. Is he on something? I mean, like a substance? He seems to be acting mildly manic.*

"What else? Anything about me?" Dale probed.

"Hmm." Dr. Lea looked him over carefully, taking her time. "You say there's something different about you? I'm looking. Just not sure. Did you color your hair?"

"Doc, you're pulling my leg."

"Yes, Dale. I did notice right away, but I thought I might offend you if I said something immediately. You're all trimmed up and nicely dressed. That's remarkable! I like it! You look good—still short of breath when you walked up to the door, but you look better while doing it. What gives? And why?" *Okay, I really don't think he's taking anything to make him this way. His manner seems to be genuine, but it's astounding.*

"I had a heart-to-heart talk with my son, Aaron. He was going to try to be here today but couldn't get off work."

"You did? That's terrific! How did that come about?"

"Well, have a seat, doc. I'll tell you." Other than the absent blue haze and the greater light in the room, Dr. Lea noted that nothing else had changed.

"I called your office the day after our last visit. Talked to Robert, the social worker. He gave me some advice about the goals of care discussion, he called it. We talked for a half hour. His advice was like yours. But when talking about the decision-maker, Robert called him the agent. We talked about my son.

"I hadn't talked with Aaron for over five years. He didn't come to his mom's funeral. We've had a running disagreement—I can't even remember now what it was about. Go figure, right?

"He, I mean Robert, the social worker, not Aaron, my son, suggested I read a book called *The Four Things that Matter Most.*[4] It would help me get a better attitude toward Aaron, he said, so we could have a talk about what you and I last talked about. Is this making any sense, Doc?"

"Oh, yes. Perfect sense, Dale. Go on—I want to hear more."

"So, once I started I couldn't put the book down. It explained in terms I could relate to and lots of real-life examples. You've read it before, right, doc?"

"Yes, I have. I heard the author speak at a conference once."

"Oh, that's cool. His four things in the book make sense, and it broke down my bad attitude toward Aaron. I went through the four steps in my head, and I wrote them out too. In order. They go: Please forgive me. I forgive you. Thank you. I love you.

"I have to say, I've never said all that to one person in my whole life. Never."

"How did that make you feel?" Dr. Lea asked. *He's not crying but smiling.*

"Good. Way down inside good. Aaron was shocked, probably like you are—but you're too nice to say so."

"True, and thanks." Dr. Lea looked straight at Dale. "You read me pretty well."

"I told you I was a good judge of character. But, anyway, like you said to me a couple weeks ago, this kind of talking will set an example for others. It helped me not to be afraid.

"Really, I'm as shocked as everyone else about how different it makes me feel. Others are noticing too. Even Hannah out there said so, didn't you?" Dale called out toward the kitchen with his head turned that way.

"Oh, yes. Big difference. He doesn't yell at me anymore and . . ."

"Okay, that's enough, Hannah. You don't have to tell the doc everything, do ya?" Dale chuckled and slapped his knee with a loud smack. "Ouch! That was harder than I meant."

"Obviously your talk with Aaron went well?"

"Yes. I won't get into all the specifics with ya, but he could see I was being straight with him. He told me how different I looked from more than five years ago, and I think he got scared. He understood what I was talking about, but he gave me no trouble about it. And he said he was okay with being my advocate. Robert called it agent—same as decision-maker, right?"

"Yes, that's right."

"We got all the way through it, all four things. We both did them. And he told me he loved me at the end. Never thought that was something I'd hear from Aaron.

"Doc, you got me tearing up. That didn't happen with Aaron, but it's hitting me as I explain it to you."

"No problem. That's normal. You're okay." She let him be for a minute, then went on,

"Where are you at with completing the document? Are you going to do it, then?"

"Oh, yeah. I'm almost done."

"Any questions about it?"

"Don't think so. Seems to be straightforward. So, people pay lawyers a lot of money to do this kind of thing?"

"Glad you're going through it. Yes, they do, but it's usually along with other legal documents like wills or estate planning—part of a package deal. It can be a good thing for people to involve their attorney; you know things can get messy. These are straightforward but do need to be properly completed. Yours might be simpler to do.

"Do you want to share with me some of your decisions?"

"I guess I can. No CPR! That's for sure—none of that chest compressing stuff. No to the kidney filtering. No to the tube feedings or whatever they call them. I want the breathing machine if the docs think I'll make it. Can they do it for a while to see how I do?"

"That's exactly what they can do. You bring up a good point: many people think that once you start it up you have to stay on it 'til you die, but that's not the case. There can be clear reasons to start and stop it; we call it withdrawal when you're going through the stopping stage.

"When they do that they make sure you remain comfortable, without any feeling of being short of breath, through the use of medicines. Most people are unconscious during that time and aren't aware of what's going on around them. So, that part wouldn't be stressing you out. And, by the way, that withdrawal can be done for other interventions like feeding tubes or dialysis."

"Feel better about that one." Dale flashed a thumbs up. "I want oxygen and antibiotics or other medications to keep me going if it looks like it might be a short illness and I can recover. If not, then I don't want them. If they're already started, it'll be okay with me to stop . . . or the other word you said. If from the start it looks like I can't make it, then don't start those things at all."

"Dale, I hear you. That's how you have to say it in your form and explain it to Aaron. Do you have a backup person for Aaron, in case he can't do it for some reason?"

"Yeah, I do. It's Hannah." The sound of breaking glass from the kitchen alarmed them both as he finished the sentence. Dr. Lea ran to the kitchen in time to help Hannah sit in a kitchen chair.

"What's wrong with Hannah?" Dale asked, trying to get up from his recliner.

"She's okay, Dale. Don't fall yourself trying to rush over here. She's fine. A dish or something broke in the sink, but she's not cut—there's no bleeding. She's sitting up fine."

Now directed to Hannah, "How are you feeling?" Dr. Lea had her stethoscope on Hannah's chest and was checking her vitals. *Pallor, sweaty, slow pulse. Probably a low BP too. A near-syncopal episode.* "She nearly fainted, but she's coming around." Dale was breathing hard as he reached the kitchen.

"That's a strong emotional reaction from Hannah to what you just said. Does that seem strange to you, Dale?" *Hannah's color is returning to normal, and her pulse is calming down.*

Her sweating is resolving. She's over it. "She's getting over it now."

"Oh, that's good. Hannah, you want me to tell the doc?"

Hannah nodded her approval.

"Doc, you see, Hannah is my adopted daughter's only child. I've raised her for probably fifteen years, along with my wife when she was alive. Her parents died in a car accident at the same time. They were both drunk, and fortunately Hannah wasn't in the car with them when it happened. We've taken care of her since. She's my caregiver now. She's paid for by the insurance company."

"That explains some things I've noticed, but this still seems like an exaggerated reaction to me."

"I know it does. Can we just leave it with that? I'm trying to protect her."

"Yes, of course," Dr. Lea agreed thoughtfully. "I don't want to harm her or make anything worse."

"It's nothing like that. She told me before, when Dr. Dryden talked about these things, that she doesn't want to be placed in any kind of decision-making role. When she's stressed she passes out."

"I see. That's called stress-induced syncope—a type of vasovagal syncope."

"Which means . . . ?"

"A simple fainting spell when she experiences stress. Has she been to a doctor for it?"

"No." Dale motioned for Dr. Lea to move to the other side of the room. "And that's what I'm trying to protect. She has a fear of doctors. She's told me she likes you and trusts you, but when it comes to herself she doesn't want anything to do with doctors."

"Well, she should really be checked out, at least on a basic level, to be sure there's nothing else going on."

"I know, doc. I get it, but she doesn't. I've tried when other things happen, like when she's sick and such, but no way. Good thing she hasn't gotten really sick." Dale made the sign of the cross.

"Are you Catholic?"

"Yeah."

"Well, me too. You continue to surprise me, Dale."

"I have to admit I don't always live out my faith. I've done my share of wandering, shall I say? What I've noticed is when I wander from the basics of my faith, then I wander in my life. It's like a mirror; if I step away from the mirror and forget what I look like, I'm not really following God and what he says. I've had good stretches, but they don't always last.

"You've heard that one before, doc?"

"I have. You're certainly deeper inside than you seemed when I was first getting to know you."

"That's my defense mechanism. Protect myself. Like I want to protect Hannah. But, hey, I heard that about the mirror, and it gives me something I can picture and relate to—helps it stick with me. When I forget what I look like, I go to God and ask for forgiveness and get back on track. When I spoke with my priest before, he told me God has no limit on forgiveness; that's another one that sticks with me. If I didn't believe that I would've given up long ago, . . . and who knows what or where I'd be now." Dale shuddered.

"Let's go back and check on Hannah in the kitchen," Dr. Lea suggested. "Put the broom away, Hannah. We'll clean up the mess. You keep resting in the chair."

"No, that's okay. I'm fine now."

"Like it's happened before?"

"Pretty much." Hannah kept on cleaning up the mess as Dr. Lea crouched down to help with the big pieces that lay there.

————

"Dale, you need to write those things out about your care, as you told me earlier. Then get Aaron to sign it with two witnesses who aren't related to you. When you've done that, you'll be done with the advance directive! Yay!"

"Good. Ready for that to be over."

"Just be sure your doctors get a copy, including me."

"Deal. See you in six weeks, doc?"

"Deal."

"The rest of the mirror story, doc, is that if someone sticks with following God's Word after that, not forgetting what they see in the mirror, then they're blessed. That's worth remembering."

"Thanks, Dale. You're convincing. See you in six weeks."

Dr. Lea walked to her car, satisfied with what she had heard and what had happened today with Dale.

14

PEARL

CUSTARD PIE

Ten Days Later

"GOOD morning, Pearl," Dr. Lea began. "You're looking much better than when I saw you last at the hospital. You heal quickly! Where's Erin? I thought she might be with you."

"Oh, no. I shooed her home a couple days ago. I'm doing fine, and she was bored. I feel back to how I was before I got sick."

"That's remarkable; that was much faster than I expected it to go for you."

"I'm glad for it," Pearl replied.

"Me too. Let's talk about your pain. What's your pain level, and how has it been?"

"It's pretty much back to the usual. In the morning I take the two acetaminophens for the milder morning pain, and then the combo stronger pain med, only one at night. It's working."

"That's good." *No rubbing of her sides this time.*

"Yes, I'm pleased," Pearl agreed. "I finished taking the antibiotics. I had a follow up culture of my urine, and it was negative. Follow up labs were back to normal too."

"Well, that's all good. Any other troubles? Fatigue changes? Bowel habits okay?"

"No other troubles, besides the fatigue. Surprisingly, it doesn't seem as bad after the bad illness I had."

"Hmm. You're probably still off the Tykitrol until you see Oncology, Right?"

"Yes, that's right." Pearl sat up a little straighter. "I didn't make the connection. You're thinking that, with my being off the Tykitrol, the fatigue is better?"

"That's my thought. Don't restart it, if you're wondering, until you see your oncologist. When is that appointment?"

"Next week or so. It's on my calendar at home. Okay, I'm thinking about it, but I'll see how I am from now 'til then. You've got me thinking, Dr. Lea," Pearl mused. "It might be a good time to try being off it and see how I feel."

"Or maybe until your next scan to see what changes there are before restarting it?"

"Maybe," Pearl reflected. "Oh, before I forget, my birthday is coming up next week, and I want to invite you over for a piece of custard pie. My recipe. It's a tradition for me. Will you come?"

"You give me the date. And if we can make it an early afternoon or right after lunch, I can probably do it."

"Okay, I'll call your office back. Hope you can make it, even if it's short."

"Yes, I hope so too." Standing now, Dr. Lea hugged Pearl.

———

"Pearl, this is the best custard pie I've ever eaten! I'm serious—this is amazing."

"Just an old-fashioned family recipe. I always use Foster's. Well, it's really Foster Clark's Custard Powder, and I use the vanilla flavor. It works perfectly every time, I must say. You can't find it everywhere, but it's around."

"Then I'll have to get Foster's. I'll look around, and, if not, I'll look online." Forks down and no crumbs left behind, Dr. Lea and Pearl sipped on their remaining Bewley's Earl Grey black tea. Pearl insisted on using the specialty imported Irish black tea, and Dr. Lea could taste why. "Well, thank you, Pearl, for the invite to share this special dessert and tea with you on your birthday. Unforgettable! Thank you. I have to go, but I wish I could stay all afternoon."

Pearl's house had been a distraction for Dr. Lea, the decor a mix of her Irish heritage and American. Comfortable and nice, but not extravagant. Dr. Lea imagined Pearl raising her family there. The family photos neatly arranged on the walls of the living room fit Pearl's motif.

"Maybe another time, then," Pearl quipped with a wink. "We forgot to make the next appointment. Shall I call your office today?"

"Oh, yes. How did I forget that? Distracted by the custard pie, probably," Dr. Lea replied with a quick tummy rub. "Let's try to go back to three months."

"Okay, I'll call in and make it today." Dr. Lea, down the front porch steps, waved back without turning, so she didn't see Pearl rubbing her sides.

Sitting up for so long was a bit much, I'd say. The ache should go away.

15

PEARL

PAIN – 3

Three Months Later

"PEARL, we made it three months from your last visit." Pearl stayed seated but leaned forward to give Dr. Lea a hug.

"Yes, indeed we did, doctor." Pearl rubbed both her sides absently, answering Dr. Lea's unvoiced question.

"I see your pain is troubling you more than it looks." Dr. Lea had certainly noticed the side rubbing but also the fact that Pearl stayed seated. "Tell me more about the pain. Give me a rating today, now at the visit. Then give me an idea of how your pain is at other times of day. I'm looking for the pattern and for any changes to it."

"Right now it's a five. I took the acetaminophen, 1000 mg., this morning. I still take the combo pain medicine at night. It works, but less well, and I'm waking up with more pain in the morning. By less well I mean that it gives me relief but doesn't last as long as it did before."

Dr. Lea noted the changes and then asked, "What about the pattern? Have you noticed any changes with the timing? Or any different features of the pain?"

"The usual pain pattern is still there, but it's more severe. If I'm late taking the night dose it'll get up to level six. Like I said, the morning is stronger than a definite four, which is about double what it used to be. I've noticed this all in the last two to three weeks.

"Then there's stronger aching when I'm up and around, even if what I'm doing isn't strenuous—like light vacuuming or laundry with some twisting and lifting movements. The pain remains in my sides. It doesn't move around. I'm not sure, but I think it's about equal on both sides. There's a strong ache and now a slight burning on the left side when it's the most severe." *I don't want her to change my medication, but maybe I should if she talks about it.*

"Pearl, I think it's time we talk about your pain medicine regimen. Before we do that, though, I want to know more about what's going on with your CML. What have they said to you about it?"

"The labs are the same: high white cell count—32,000 last time. The platelets are down to 25,000, and the blood count is 10. Is that the hemoglobin number?" Pearl asked.

"Right, that's the hemoglobin. Normal is around 14 grams, plus or minus a couple grams. Your white count is up some, and your platelets are down from normal ranges. What about the latest scans?"

"Yes, well, the lymph nodes deep in the back of my abdomen, they're slowly enlarging, and the spleen is also enlarging. The liver did, too, but not as much, the doc said."

"Are you bruising or bleeding more than usual? You haven't had big problems with that so far."

"Slightly, I'd say. Nothing major."

"What do you think about all this? Did Dr. Ludlow talk about it?"

"Yes, he said it meant progression of the disease. We had just restarted the Tykitrol about a month ago, before the scans and blood tests were done."

"That makes it hard to know what to do," Dr. Lea reflected, anticipating the discussion of the TKI.

"Exactly. How did you know?" Pearl winked. "I was going to ask for your opinion on a couple matters I talked with them about. Is that all right?"

"Yes, for sure—please do."

"Since restarting the Tykitrol my tiredness is worse—it's more noticeable to the point I've got to slow down at home. I'm leaving dishes in the sink overnight. I vacuum only once a week, and then I have to split it up to two days with rests between rooms. I'm shopping less, and Erin is helping me with that too.

"Then there's the next steps idea Dr. Ludlow gave me to think about. I want to hear what you think about it." Pearl didn't hesitate here but continued quickly, "He explained that my previous treatment with Tykitrol and then the other TKIs I didn't tolerate a few years back doesn't leave a lot of other choices for the leukemia. He's concerned the disease is becoming more resistant, and with my high-risk genetic profile, combined with the Philadelphia chromosome, there's a risk the CML will convert into an acute form of leukemia. He didn't give me a timeframe, and I didn't ask. That last part scares me the most."

Again without hesitation, Pearl continued her lengthy explanation before launching into her questions. "He said there's an intense form of treatment for my situation, but I'd need infusion twice a day for two weeks to get it started. I'd have to have another bone marrow test. You know how I love those!" Wink.

"So, I'm wondering about your thoughts on the disease progression," Dr. Lea began. "Did the stopping of Tykitrol contribute to it progressing? What do you think of undergoing the bone marrow test and then this advanced I.V. treatment?"

"Well, he described the side effects—and they don't sound like fun; 99–100% have side effects, with some of them serious and life-threatening, like bleeding and stroke. Not even half the people who start the study finish, but for those who do—mostly younger patients who are healthy otherwise—the results are very good at slowing down the disease."

"Pearl, there's a lot to talk about. You're sounding more and more medical. But before I get started sharing my opinion, I want to ask you a question. Do the next steps—the testing and this very serious treatment—fit with what your goals for yourself? You've been doing so well for so long that all of this hasn't been part of our discussions; we've mainly touched on your symptoms and on updating your advance directive.

"The very slow progression of CML over years of time makes it that way. So, my question is really, with what you know about what Dr. Ludlow described, does the idea of going down that path give you a sense of peace or satisfaction, with no regret? Is it consistent with your goals or wishes for your life, or does it cross the line and make you uncomfortable with the thought that it may be more than you want to do?

"Would you regret taking those steps, considering the risks, if something went badly for you as a result? Or, to put it another way, would you be at peace without even finding out what the testing and treatment could bring you?"

"Yes, I see what you mean, Dr. Lea. You know how to get to the heart of the matter. I appreciate your direct but gentle approach with me; you don't make me scared talking about it at all. I wish Erin could have been here.

"Honestly." Pearl paused now. "What . . . what I'm about to say I've never spoken out loud before, except one time when I was praying to the Lord. I still pray—my Catholic upbringing stays strong in me—but now he seems more personal and less stern as I call out to him in my distress. I've been reading in the book of Psalms in the Bible, and that has comforted me. I'm sure you understand what I mean.

"Let me get back to your question now. When I answer the question, taking into account what I think is best for me and not what others might want me to do, my answer is a clear no. I don't want those tests—they hurt and are uncomfortable, and for what reason?— since I don't believe I want to try that aggressive I.V. treatment Dr. Ludlow described."

Dr. Lea paused here. She wanted to give Pearl an opportunity to mentally confirm what her heart was telling her would be okay, and to confirm that it would be okay for her to say these words to someone else.

Dr. Lea had learned this approach from other instances when she had found herself blurting out something just to fill the empty space. She had felt at those times that the emptiness of space was uncomfortable to allow, fearing that emotions might bubble up from the patient, causing Dr. Lea to feel the same ones in herself—then what would she do? She had learned from such experiences to slow it down and let the quiet time have its way. *It works; I'll let Pearl have her moment here.*

———

"For your pain you described to me today, Pearl, I'd like to start a stronger medication that has no acetaminophen in it. It'll be strong pain medicine, another type of opioid. Now, don't be alarmed by the one I'm picking for you to take—it's morphine. We're going to start you on roughly an equivalent amount of opioid in each dose, and you can take it every four hours as needed.

"This will help us find out how much you need in a day to get comfortable. It'll take several days to find this out, and we might need to make dose adjustments to get there, but to begin with the dose will be roughly equal to what your body is used to taking from the strong pain medicine.

"Eventually over the next couple weeks we'll see how much you need to get your pain to a level that's comfortable for you and then start you on a long-acting form of morphine so that you won't have to take it as often. The long-acting pills last from eight to twelve hours. You'll have the short-acting form of morphine still on hand for any pain in between the long-acting tablets.

"This dosing schedule is how it's done, and it's safe and effective. It will get you to your goal of better pain control. You won't need to use the combo pain pills at all, so you can get rid of those at the pharmacy. And you can still take the acetaminophen if you need something for lower levels of pain, like a two or a three.

"We'll give you written instructions to have on hand. We'll send in the prescription for you, and you don't need to start it until the morning after you get it. Keep track by writing down how many of the short-acting tabs you're taking in a day—by that, I mean I twenty-four hours. So, when you start in the morning, the twenty-four hours will end the following morning. This is important because we'll ask you to let us know the number of these short-acting tabs you're taking so we can see how you're doing and know how to make changes if we need to.

"The morphine has similar side effects to the pills you've taken before. You already have a bowel regimen that's working for you. If you experience nausea or vomiting or excessive drowsiness or tiredness or find yourself sleeping more, let us know about that too. What we've just talked about will all be in the written information we give you, in case you need to review. The pharmacy may give you information too.

"Does that all make sense? We'll be calling to see how you're doing with the medicine and have you back sooner too. You can always call us. Someone is always on duty.

"Now, you've just finished a short course in opioid pharmacology," Dr. Lea quipped.

"Yes, I think I get it. I can always call. I think I'll ask Erin to stay with me for a couple days, at least to see how I handle it. We've done that before with other medications."

"You'll be calling Dr. Ludlow to talk with him about your decision on next steps?"

"Yes, I'll call him tomorrow."

"Do you think it would be helpful if we had a family meeting with you, your son, and your daughter about your decision?"

"Let me talk with them first and see how they handle it. It may not be necessary."

"Okay, that's fine. Let's meet again in ten to fourteen days. The palliative care nurse will be calling you in two or three days to see how you're doing and answer any questions you may have. Pearl, this may seem like a lot to digest, but it's routine operation for us; we'll help you through it.

"I want to add that, if it all goes well, we can maybe change the morphine to a long-acting form, joined with the short-acting, for smoother pain control. We'll explain that to you if that looks like what we'll recommend. Okay?"

"No problem. I trust you, Dr. Lea."

Hugs.

16

PEARL and DALE

PALLIATIVE CARE SUMARY – 4

YOU are beginning to see how palliative care helps patients. A detailed approach that examines the symptoms and problems caused by the patient's serious illness and how it impacts their life sometimes also involves family members.

When family members or caregivers are involved, especially if they are not related to the family, family meetings can be helpful at important times throughout the illness. These allow everyone to hear the same information, which is often complicated and requires time for questions and deeper discussions. This also lets the doctor and other team members meet the family, sometimes for the first time, and observe how they interact and get along.

This can be insightful for the clinical team for understanding which decisions about treatment options to offer or when to think about stopping them. It's especially important to make changes in treatment when the illness is more rapidly progressing, as these changes can affect how long someone might live. For more advanced diseases, progression might necessitate a referral to hospice if the prognosis qualifies the patient for hospice care. The Medicare Hospice Benefit regulations state that the applicable patient life expectancy at the point of referral must be six months or less. This standard is also followed by other insurance and Medicaid plans.

In my companion book *Hope in Hospice* I explain that two doctors must both determine that someone is eligible for hospice care. Additionally, the patient must have a terminal illness and must choose to receive hospice services. This usually means stopping medical treatments that aim to extend life and instead focusing on ways to make and keep the patient comfortable. This allows the terminal condition to run its natural course.

While having a DNAR (Do Not Attempt Resuscitation) code status isn't required when entering hospice care, it's definitely a good idea to discuss this option now that two physicians (one being the patient's primary care doctor and the other the hospice doctor) concur that the serious illness is terminal.

There is, however, an alternate course of action from further disease progression to terminal status. Sometimes a patient receiving palliative care may be stable, their care goals for this level of care may have been achieved, and the primary attending physician can continue the medical treatment without needing the ongoing help of the palliative care team. This usually happens when a patient has been sent to palliative care mainly to talk about goals instead of managing symptoms.

Once the goals are set and plans have been created to reach them, the patient has successfully accomplished their goals. It is highly recommended that talking about care goals results in completing advance directives, also known as power of attorney in healthcare. In this way the decision-maker can be officially named, assigned their role, and legally recognized.

The form requires the right signatures and witnesses. Each state is responsible for these documents, as they are not governed by federal regulations, so the details will vary from state to state. It's important to understand the requirements of the state in which the patient resides. A notary public and/or witnesses will be needed.

It is advisable to check with the person's doctor's office or attorney, if they have one, to help complete these documents, although the patient and family can opt to fill out the forms themselves or use templates to help them complete this step on their own. If they hire a lawyer the process is usually handled in conjunction with formulating wills and planning estates.

Advanced palliative care pain management

Controlling pain is important and is a main focus for palliative care teams to evaluate and manage. The members have advanced training and skills to identify the type of pain the person is experiencing and to create effective ways to manage it. This is especially true since there are different types of pain the body feels, each with its own features and each responding to a different approach for treatment.

Pearl was feeling a change in pain as her condition progressed. Some of it was her usual pain, which was getting worse, but some a different kind of pain. This necessitated a change in approach to treating the pain that involved not just changing the amount of medication but also using different types of medication that would work better to alleviate the new pain. Strong pain medicine, which I will keep referring to as opioids, is often used. However, there are non-opioid medicines that can treat certain kinds of pain or make opioids more effective, often allowing for a reduction in the amount of opioids needed.

The palliative care team has the experience and desire to help with symptoms. While palliative care team members do not have to be certified to work in this field, today most of them have taken extra training in a specific area of expertise. This means that after a doctor has completed their specialty training (after becoming a family doctor, internist, anesthesiologist, surgeon, or emergency physician, for example), they will spend an extra year in a subspecialty training program for palliative care and hospice. At the end of this program they will take a board exam to become certified in that specialty field. Nurses and social workers can earn their certification by passing a test.

Many primary care doctors and specialists recognize that the palliative care team plays an important role in managing symptoms. In cases of serious illness, the first or second course of treatment may not work well, and the advanced skills and knowledge of palliative care specialists are often required to create a more complex treatment plan. This may involve less common medicines or a combination of medications requiring additional expertise to prescribe safely and effectively.

Infrequently a procedure is suggested to help lessen or manage the pain or other symptoms. Most palliative care doctors don't perform these procedures themselves, but some pain specialists who work in palliative care do.

The most common symptom of advanced disease is pain, and the most common type of pain is categorized as malignant pain; this is pain related to cancer, whether from the effects of the disease itself or from the treatment. The palliative care team concentrates on the pain from the serious illness, not on the totality of the pain the patient may be experiencing. I will carefully explain.

One common type of pain is arthritis, or pain in the joints. This kind of pain usually isn't the main concern for the palliative care team because it doesn't result from a serious illness. If the palliative care team is helping a patient with heart failure, and the only pain the patient has is from arthritis, the team will leave the handling of the pain to the patient's primary care doctor or other specialists, like an arthritis doctor or an orthopedist.

Another common issue is chronic pain. This is a completely different, complex condition that requires expert doctors and a team of medical professionals for proper management. The palliative care team will focus on treating the pain from the serious illness, but they won't directly address pain from other, unrelated conditions. This can be difficult to sort out, but it is important. The palliative care doctor and the pain specialist will need to work together, each in their own field of expertise, to determine the best way to treat the different types of pain a patient is experiencing. Some of the medicines I would use for treating serious illness pain are not used for chronic pain.

Additional information on topics related to pain is covered in the Appendix. There I review the topics of chronic pain, cancer pain, other types of pain, and ancillary medications for assistance in relieving pain. How the palliative care provider adjusts pain medications is explained there, and I describe in more detail specialized types of pain and the interventional approach to its treatment.

Shortness of breath/breathlessness

Breathlessness, no matter the cause—such as long-term lung or heart disease, cancer, or serious kidney or liver problems—is treated in palliative care in much the same way it is in regular medical care, especially when the initial focus of the medical providers is on the disease itself. For people with long-lasting lung problems, this means using inhalers, nebulizers, oxygen, and other devices that don't require surgery to help with breathing.

In palliative care for these conditions, these treatments are continued or ordered if they haven't been used previously. Most of the time patients referred for palliative care already have these treatments in place, however, for their advanced symptoms. These care regimens will be continued or modified, and if the patient does not follow the instructions they will be encouraged to take or use the medicine or utilize treatments.

It is only after these steps that treatment focused on palliative medicine is considered. The same applies to severe heart disease. The treatment for the specific disease is continued first, after which other options are considered. The same approach applies when cancer-causing and serious kidney or liver diseases are leading to the shortness of breath: care begins by concentrating on the methods specific to those diseases.

After the lung disease-specific methods are used, if the symptoms continue to be troublesome palliative care might suggest other methods or medicines to reach desired levels of comfort. Most of the time this entails the use of opioids for symptom relief. Opioid use to alleviate pain is a general treatment, meaning that it can work for a variety of conditions without targeting a specific mechanism of the underlying disease.

Understanding how opioids help with shortness of breath explains why they are used. The exact way this works isn't fully understood, but it is thought that a few different processes help relieve breathlessness. First, for the causes related to the respiratory or breathing system, opioids are believed to affect the sensors in the body that detect the feeling of not being able to breathe properly.

Opioids acting on these receptors provide relief for this feeling. They usually work fast, often in the same amount of time required for pain relief. If the medicine is taken by mouth it will take twenty to forty minutes for it to work, but if it is administered through an intravenous (IV) line it can start working in just seconds to minutes; this is because it goes directly into the bloodstream and reaches the receptors much more quickly.

When medication is taken by mouth it has to pass through the lining of the stomach and intestines before entering the bloodstream. From there it travels through the liver and then into the general circulation, which carries it around the body so it can act on various receptors and produce its effects. Opioids are believed to work in the same manner for treating shortness of breath caused by other issues or by cancer.

When opioids are used to treat pain related to heart disease, there is a similar effect on the receptors but also another, more specific circulatory effect. The opioid slows down the blood returning to the heart, which lowers the pressure on a weak heart and reduces congestion in the lungs, where blood takes in oxygen and releases carbon dioxide. The opioid regimen works very well for this condition.

The methods for administering the medication in this situation are the same as for the relief of other pain, and the same side effects can occur when it is used for these conditions. The long-lasting versions can also be effective if the circumstances are suitable for opioid use. There are different reasons for using or not using them, and it is up to the doctor and the patient to discuss them, as mentioned elsewhere in the book.

———

While the patient is under the care of the palliative care team, the physician and other providers are looking for the correct ongoing course for them. There are three choices: continue in the program, discharge from the program, or transition to hospice care. This evaluation does not always involve a formal process by the clinician but is based on a clinical feeling of how the patient is doing over a period of time.

If there is ongoing need for clinical intervention and symptom management, the patient clearly continues to be eligible for the services. If, however, the patient enters a period of stability in terms of their condition or even improves, planning for discharge back to the full care of the primary care provider and specialists may be suitable. If there is progressive deterioration and the sense of a life-limiting prognosis being appropriate, a hospice referral is considered.

This is not to say that these kinds of joint decisions happen with every patient encountered. The process is generally less formal than that. But as the palliative care team notices changes or improvement, any of the members may bring up for consideration the possibility of plan changes or development.

Such a change in approach involves careful discussion with the patient. Delivering news—either bad or good—is a skill to be learned; there is a right way and a wrong way to do either. This is an important reason for specialized learning programs to teach and assess learners in gaining expertise and a level of comfort in this kind of advanced communication. This is an example of the palliative care clinician's specialty "procedures" of communication.

17

DALE

CONCLUSIONS

Six Weeks Later

DR. Lea completed her usual physical assessment of Dale and then settled in for the history taking and discussion.

"Dale, your exam remains at your baseline. No changes. You're taking your usual medications, inhalers, nebulizers, and oxygen. Is that right?"

"Right, doc. And you noticed no return of the blue haze here. I've completely quit the smokes." Applause from the kitchen from Hannah.

"That's good news! Have you had any sudden shortness of breath feelings or episodes?"

"None at all," Dale replied with evident satisfaction.

"Good news with that too. Other symptoms or troubles you're having?"

"None that you don't know about already, doc."

"That brings me to our discussion from last time about your advance directive. Did you get signatures and witnesses?"

"That I did. All set. I have a copy for you to take. My doctors' offices all have a copy too."

"Perfect."

"This brings me to the next topic—I hope you're ready for it."

"Go ahead, doc. I know what it is. I've been expecting it."

"You never cease to surprise me, Dale. Will that make it easier to talk about?"

"Maybe—we'll see." Hannah made an intentional throat-clearing noise in the kitchen. "You might as well come in here, Hannah," Dale invited. She complied.

"Right, so let's talk about it, then. You've been in our palliative care service for over three years. And since I've been visiting you we've accomplished quite a lot. That was built on the success of Dr. Dryden to that point. Agree?"

"Yes. I'm with you, doc."

"I believe the palliative care program has accomplished all that it needed to with you. I hope you agree with that too. Your condition has stabilized. No hospital admits or even emergency visits for a few years now. Your medication regimen is unchanged, and you're tolerating it.

"You've had no severe bad breathing episodes in months, and you're compliant with everything we've asked of you. In addition, you've quit smoking and are more alert. You're still weak and still with severe lung disease, of course. None of that has gone away . . . "

"You don't need to remind me of that, doc. I am very winded, as you know. The rest of what you said is all true."

"Plus, you've talked with your son—restored the relationship with him. You've thought about your medical care goals, wrote them down, finished the advance directive documents, and given them to your doctors and to us. Thank you."

Dale nodded politely.

"After outlining all of this, I think the palliative care team has helped you figure out your goals and made sure your current care and future care wishes match those goals. And you're satisfied with your quality of life. Is that true, Dale?"

"Yes, it is. Just as you said."

"So, I'm proposing we give it one month, and if your condition doesn't change or show any reason for us to expect it to change dramatically in the coming months, I think the palliative care team can sign off your care service."

"I think I understand, but what does that all mean?" Dale queried.

"We'll communicate with your primary care physician and lung specialist, letting them know we're stepping back from direct involvement with your care. We'll give them a full report, so you can be sure they're comfortable with the current plan of care you're under and that they're willing to take that over from us. From then on they will order any equipment, medications, or supplies you may need. including your oxygen. So far so good?" Dr. Lea asked, pausing to wait for a reply.

"I'm with you, doc," Dale agreed.

"We will begin to communicate with them after today's visit. We'll let them know about the one-month plan to discharge you from our care because of all the reasons we just talked about. I'll come back one more time in a month to check on you and review the final plan with you in detail. You can ask questions. I want you to be totally comfortable with all of this, Dale. That's important to me."

"Got it. Deal, doc."

"Glad to hear it. Do you have any questions at this time?"

"No."

"Okay, then that will be the plan."

"Doc, how's your mirror?" Dale could see her puzzled look. "You know, when you look away from the mirror, do you remember what you look like?"

"Oh, yes. That's right. Yes, thanks for the reminder. You got me on that one, Dale," Dr. Lea assented. Dale smiled.

18

PEARL

PAIN – 4

Twelve Days Later

"DR. Lea, how are you doing today?" Pearl asked before the doctor could get into the door of the exam room.

"Pearl, well—how's your pain with the different pain medication, switching from your combo pain med to the morphine? I know the nurse has been talking with you every few days to track your symptoms and medicine effects." *Pearl looks a lot more comfortable this time around. I hope it's all going well for her.*

"Doctor, I couldn't be more pleased. I'm just plain happy, I guess. The pain is definitely under control. In very little time I only needed the pain medicine every four hours, with rarely anything in between. No trouble with nausea or constipation—the same regimen is working well for me still.

"I don't miss the old pain medicine at all. I'm so glad to have switched. The nurse was great calling me every couple days. I did have some extra tiredness at the start, but that quickly went away. No other trouble. I wasn't confused or anything like that. Erin stayed with me for three nights, and she and I were satisfied. Your nurse felt it was safe too."

"Yes, she told me that. And we were able to add the long-acting form for you as well. That's on a twelve-hour schedule. I'm pleased with that."

"Yes, it all went perfectly. I had no trouble at all."

"Great. You can still have the short-acting tablet to have on hand if you need something in between. Do you recall that this was our plan when we changed your pain medicine around?"

"Yes. That's perfectly fine. Thank you."

"Now, let's talk about the other questions we discussed last time. Do you remember, Pearl?"

"My, yes, I sure do. I asked some tough questions, and you came back with the big question of what my goals were for treatment and testing. I told you I wanted none of the advanced testing—the bone marrow test or that I.V. treatment with such severe side effects. I'm sticking with that, no doubt whatsoever." *She's nodding in agreement, so I will continue, but I'm not sure she'll agree with what I have to say.*

"I discussed all of that with Dr. Ludlow," Pearl went on, "and he actually seemed relieved by the choice I made. I think he felt he had to tell me all my options . . . but, anyway, he accepted my choice. However, since I'm feeling so much better again, I told him I want to stay on the Tykitrol." Pearl looked down momentarily, then back up just in time. *I've never seen Dr. Lea tap her finger on her cheek as she sits there looking at me. Is she mad? Or disappointed in me? Or thinking about what she's going to say next. Well, it doesn't matter. It's my choice, and I've got to go with what I think is best.*

"Pearl, I'll have to say you surprised me this time." Dr. Lea looked straight into Pearl's eyes. "But I'm not disappointed. First, I'm very glad you spoke with Dr. Ludlow about his input, and I totally agree. I'm pleased as well that you're sticking with your decision to forego the bone marrow test and the I.V. treatment we talked about last time.

"You know, it's so easy sometimes as a patient to just go along with the next 'thing' a doctor might bring up or recommend. It's much tougher and takes courage to go against the flow, put the brakes on, and make the decision that's right for you and your goals. So, I congratulate you! I really do.

"Second, with regard to the Tykitrol choice you're making, you know my thoughts professionally about it, but I like that you're consistent in your decision. I also believe, Pearl, that when it's the right time to stop it you'll be convinced of that and will have no regret about discontinuing. You'll have peace about it at that time—that's a worthwhile goal in itself." Pearl nodded. *No words.*

"Pearl, can I bring up another topic to discuss? One you must face at some point—it has to do with your prognosis. Is it okay to talk about it?"

"Yes, you know it is. You know me by now, Dr. Lea."

"Yes, but I want your permission." *I sure wish Erin were here today to hear this with her mom.*

"Well then, you have it. I've got a hunch you wish Erin was here with me today."

"You're reading my mind. That's true. Let me ask a question first. What has Dr. Ludlow said about your prognosis? Has he given you any updates with the changes going on? He's the kind of doctor you're probably going to have to ask to get this kind of information."

"He didn't give me any specifics on that. But as we talked he made it seem like I'm on the verge of quick changes when they do happen. He just didn't give a specific time frame."

"How do you feel about that, Pearl?" *She seems rather*

calm and matter of fact about this, considering the degree of
uncertainty on the timeline.

"I've been through so much, Dr. Lea, that I'm settled with it
at this point. I have renewed my faith commitment, so thoughts
about after death don't bother me." Pearl shrugged. "I can say
that now, knowing that how I feel may change when I know
it's closer. As I see it, pursuing what gives me spiritual peace
now will strengthen me to handle what comes next. Then,
with what palliative care has done for me, when I'm handed
off, so to speak, to the hospice care team I know they'll carry
on caring for me in the best way possible.

"I hope my family can see it this way—I can't control them,
but if they see me handling it well I hope that legacy, or more
like that memory, will stick with them and comfort them. I
see this as a final gift to them. I've made my peace with everyone. I've cleared up any past concerns and made it all right
with them; whether something was my fault or theirs doesn't
matter anymore.

"I've chosen for my part to overlook and forgive. I've told
everyone I love them. What time I have left I want to fully
embrace. That's why I chose to continue the Tykitrol. I think
staying on it is at least slightly slowing down the timetable,
and as long as I feel as good as I do I see that as a gain." Another shrug.

"Pearl, that's a whole lot of deep thought and perspective.
Thanks for sharing it with me."

"You asked me, so that's my answer. Thank *you*."

"You've made your case, and it makes sense. I see no need
or path to try convincing you otherwise; let's stick with that.
When there is evidence of further progression on scans and
with any overall changes in your condition and functioning,
these will give us a sense of a decreasing prognosis with a

direction of hospice at that point. Do you agree with that, Pearl?"

"Yes."

"I hate to bring it up, but your fatigue—how is it?" *She's rubbing her left side and the front of her left hip this time.*

"It's gradually worsening. For now it's an acceptable tradeoff. I can see, though, that when it interferes with activities that might be motivation to stop Tykitrol." *There she is, tapping her finger on her cheek again. What did I say this time?*

"Is your pain level comfortable for you right now? You're rubbing the area of your left hip; I don't remember that from before."

"Well, the strong, aching pain on the odd occasion spreads like a zinger around my side and toward my groin, in front of my left hip—but that's not daily."

"Right. Well, let me check you over." Dr. Lea examined Pearl, noting definite enlargement of the spleen on the left—possibly the source of her left-sided ache that was shooting into the left groin. The only other change noted was a small lymph node on the right side of her neck, at the base near her clavicle. Her heart, lungs, and the rest of her abdominal exam showed no change. Pearl continued to have small superficial bruises on her skin, and especially on her arms and hands. No edema in the legs was noted.

"Pearl, let's have you back in six weeks. Make sure you don't run out of your medications. Call us with any concerns."

"Okay, Dr. Lea. I'll see you then . . . if not before."

Hugs.

19

PEARL

HOSPITAL

Three Weeks Later

"LEA, this is getting to be a habit for you, coming into the hospital. Another PC patient to see?" Dr. Troy Needmore called out to her as she came around the corner from the physician/medical staff entrance of Community General Hospital. She could feel as much as hear his arrogant undertones as he called out from down the hall.

"Hi, Dr. Needmore. This is a coincidence. I come to the hospital twice, and both times I run into you. Yes, on my way to the ICU to see the same patient."

"Love to chit chat with you, but I've got to run to the board meeting." He pronounced those last three words as slowly and pretentiously as the title of the meeting sounded but sped by her afterward, the tapping of his shoes fading from around another corner. She was glad to have him exit quickly to lessen the obligatory interaction.

Dr. Lea reached the critical care unit without further interruption. She greeted the nurses and other staff on the unit long enough to not appear in a hurry to enter the patient room. When she did she found Erin in the chair and Pearl with her eyes closed, like a scene repeated from a couple of months earlier.

"Here we are again," Dr. Lea reflected to Erin as much as to anyone else; Pearl's nurse and patient care assistant were in the room too. They were charting, updating the whiteboard, and removing an untouched food tray. Dr. Lea didn't recognize either one of them, not did Pearl acknowledge Dr. Lea. *That's a change.*

Dr. Lea noted slow and unlabored breathing, with oxygen tubing protruding from Pearl's nostrils. I.V. fluid and a unit of packed red cells for transfusion were infusing her arm's I.V. catheter site. Pearl's skin and membranes revealed extreme pallor.

"Yes, here we are again," Erin replied reluctantly. She put down her phone and stood up across the bed from Dr. Lea.

"Doctor, I'm Meghan, Pearl's nurse this shift. I'm sorry, but you just missed the rounding team and the hospital palliative care doctor by about thirty minutes. You probably don't recognize me, but I was orienting when you were graduating from your fellowship. It's been a while."

"Thank you, Meghan. I don't remember but do appreciate the information. Was this the PC team's first visit to see Pearl?"

"I don't believe so; they saw her yesterday, which was the day after admission. Do you want me to pull up their notes? I have her chart opened right now, but I'm leaving her room to go next door."

"No, thanks. You go ahead and do your next tasks or whatever you have going on next room over. I can quickly log in and get to her chart. Thank you, though." Meghan closed down her chart session and left the room.

Erin began talking immediately as the nurse left. "I called the doctor and got her to the hospital as quickly as I noticed changes, and she still got very sick very quickly. Does that mean anything?"

"Without having looked in her chart yet, in general I would say yes—it does mean something, probably that her body systems as a whole, meaning all together, are functioning more poorly than they were before. I would expect she'll recover more slowly too."

"You think she will recover, then? No one has said much to me. The palliative care doctor was a little vague, but he said he was new in his fellowship and would be talking to his attending, I think he called him."

"Right, that sounds about right for a new fellow," Dr. Lea observed. "Their opinions are still forming. We have an excellent training team. I mean, they have an excellent team. I graduated from this same program, so I still sometimes call it "we" when I talk about it." Erin nodded. Pearl stirred slightly, moving her arm with the IV catheter inserted.

Dr. Lea added, "The PC team will make sure her pain medications are managed and keep her comfortable too.

"She's getting blood this time, so her red cell counts must be severely low. This is part of the CML effects on her bone marrow, plus she tends to leak blood even if it's not visible possibly in her urine or intestines. The amount you see under her skin, though, looks disturbing since it spreads out under her thin skin—it's not enough to form a large hematoma collection, like in a ball shape"—here Dr. Lea used her hands to form a round shape the size of a softball—"to make a big difference in her blood counts. She's on the same antibiotic regimen. It looks like cultures will be back tomorrow, and they can focus their selection better after knowing those results. Her heart is handling the stress on her body and reacting like it should. That's why her heart rate is up over 100 beats per minute.

"Her blood pressure has improved—it already had two days ago, and that's very good. Although she is very sick and her organs are weaker, they're still working, and she hasn't been as dehydrated as before. Her sepsis wasn't as bad as the last time. That's all because of how quickly you jumped at getting her to the hospital.

"Her kidneys are not as bad as in the last hospitalization, either—that's good too. So, all in all it could be worse, and there's every reason at this point to expect her to recover. I'm not sure how quickly or how long it will take for her to get back to her best, though. Her primary critical care team will keep you updated throughout the course." Erin's attention did not waver during this longer explanation.

"Thanks, doctor." Erin was uncharacteristically quiet.

Dr. Lea turned to the computer screen and read beyond the lab and microbiology results. She looked at the CT scans of the abdomen and chest, indicating changes in Pearl's spleen and deep abdominal lymph nodes. And the lymph nodes in the neck were just visible at the top of the uppermost image. The peripheral blood smear showed questionable early blasts (immature cells that look like cancer in this situation) with recommended bone marrow to confirm. *I know what Pearl would say about that. She chose not to tell Erin about all of these; since she didn't ask, that's a fair guess.*

Logging out of the electronic record for Pearl, Dr. Lea announced, "I'm not going to wake her this time. I'll be back in a day or two, and hopefully she'll be more awake or even alert.

"Be sure to ask questions for what you want to know from the clinical teams—that means her critical care team, her palliative care team, and the specialists." Erin nodded.

"Thank you," Erin responded.

Dr. Lea made it to the staff elevators, with the doors opening just as she arrived. But, hesitating before she stepped on, she heard her name called from a distance. She stopped, the elevator doors closed without her getting in, and she peeked back around the corner. There, speeding up to meet her, was Erin!

"Dr. Lea!" Erin called out. "Oh, good, I caught you! I know I'm not supposed to be down this hallway to your elevators," she looked over her shoulder as she strode forward, "but I followed you out of the room. I stopped, and then when I saw you go through the access door there," Erin pointing backward now, "I saw I could make it through the door to follow you. I hope you don't mind."

"No, not at all. What's on your mind, Erin?" *I think I know. I wish I'd brought it up in the room before leaving. That was my responsibility.* "Please, we can sit on these benches right here." Dr. Lea gestured for Erin to sit next to her.

"Thank you. I feel like something is missing, and I'm not sure if it's just me being paranoid—or maybe *suspicious* is the right word. Everyone is all business with me. The doctor in training didn't seem certain, and I felt like you were being so businesslike you might have been holding something back from me. Go ahead, you can tell me anything you have to say. I want to hear it. I already have a feeling, anyway, but I want to hear from you."

"Erin." Dr. Lea averted her eyes and drew a slightly deeper breath before she continued, "I'm glad you came to find me. I do have more to say. I wasn't sure you were prepared to hear it, and, to be perfectly honest, I wasn't ready myself so say it." *Lea, keep it together—you're the professional here. Slow, steady. C'mon, you know what's best for Pearl.*

Erin, puzzled, looked more intent now that she sat face-to-face with Dr. Lea on the bench. Erin could see that the doctor was trying to quell her emotions.

"Yes, you see, I've tried to be honest with your mother, but she is so insistent about how she's doing. I get a sense she covers up her symptoms and appears better than she really feels—the Irish stoic temperament, I believe. I think I've been getting somewhere with that, but her CML is speeding up, and it appears to be transforming into an acute crisis at some point soon." Dr. Lea paused, taking another deep breath. "I can't—well, no one can predict the timing—but I believe that, based on labs, her recurrent infection with sepsis, and her worsening symptoms it's getting close to happening. May I continue?"

Erin nodded with her head down.

"When the transformation comes—I'll explain that term in a second—" Dr. Lea went on, "things will change quickly. So, *from this episode* I think she has a good chance to recover, like I just said in her room. But I am concerned beyond that.

"I'm going to jump ahead here and say that I feel like we're missing out on the opportunity for hospice to help her. Yes, she's still at home, and she may recover fairly well from this incident, but we're close to the transformation moment—I mean, she's close to the CML transformation to AML, and without aggressive attempts to control it, which she has told me strongly at least twice she doesn't want, it's best to get the right kind of help. And the kind of help I mean is hospice. May I keep going?"

Erin was crying now, with repeat dabs of her eyes with a tissue. "I've seen this happen to others before. For me, let me tell you, it's personal. This same sort of scenario—not exactly the same, of course—happened to my mom. She was deteriorating from her Parkinson's but would recover just to have another setback in several weeks or a few months . . . each time not getting fully back to where she'd been. I wished hospice had been brought in sooner.

"Remember, hospice is for six months or less of life expectancy, not just for the last hours or days or weeks of life. Six months. For my mom it was only for two and a half weeks. Way too short. I don't want that to happen to yours."

"Is that why you went into this specialty, the palliative care and hospice? I mean, considering your mother's story you just told me?"

"It was part of the reason, yes."

"You've struggled with getting Mom to accept her condition; I get that—we all get that." Erin chuckled slightly. "This is your specialty, and you're a good communicator. I can tell you are, and that it's important to you. I suspect our moms must be alike in that way. Does that help you in this line of work?"

"I suppose so, yes. Getting back to your mom's case, how does one that know that the downward trajectory of a person's advanced serious illness is the final declining slope? And is that the optimal time for hospice? Honestly, I don't always know. I hope that, with even more experience during my practice, I'll gain more expertise over time. I guess that's why they call it *practice*, right?" Dr. Lea couldn't resist using the worn-out cliché; it seemed to fit.

"I plan to see your mom in a couple days. Then I'll follow up with her in clinic within a couple weeks of discharge and talk about it then." Dr. Lea touched Erin's shoulder.

"Thanks, I'd like you to do that. Not that I want it to come to this personally, but I know that's how she'd want it to be."

"I've been taking care of your mom for thirteen months, at least, maybe going on fifteen. She has lived within the range of her CML with her high-risk genetics and her prior history of breast cancer treatments very likely contributing to it. She would want me to be frank with her about her condition and general sense of her direction. Are you going to come with her to the appointment?"

"No, I think she would rather talk to you alone and then tell Patrick and me."

The elevator door opened and closed, with no one getting off or on.

Erin rose and announced, "I think I'll go back to her room now. Thanks for taking the time to explain more to me. That helps me."

"I'm glad you found me. I should have told you more back there in the room but found it difficult at the moment. I hope you understand."

"I do. Thanks." Erin turned as the elevator door opened for Dr. Lea.

———

"Pearl, I hear I caught you just before moving off the critical care floor to the regular floor. That's terrific news!" Dr. Lea enthused, stepping into the patient room.

"Hi, Dr. Lea. Yes, it's moving day today. I heard you were here the other day. I have no recollection of that at all."

"No worries. You were pretty sick, and I wasn't going to wake you up. I spoke with Erin and answered a few of her questions. How are you feeling?"

"Fair, I'd say. Tired, but that's all. I'm feeling a little bit hungry, actually."

"That's a good sign of your body recovering. How about pain?"

"It's good today. I mean, I'm stiff from the luxury mattress on this bed, but otherwise it's okay."

"Good. They're giving you the latest pain regimen with the morphine, and I'm glad it's still working. Have you been out of bed? Beyond the bedside recliner?"

"Yes, I have. Down the hallway to the halfway point and then back to my room."

"That's great. Any questions for me, Pearl? I don't mean to be rushing, but I see they're out in the hall with transportation to your next room."

"No questions I can think of right now. Glad to have you visit and we could talk," Pearl said.

"Okay, I'll have my office call you after you're discharged to set up your next visit at the clinic. Sound good?"

"Sure does. See you then."

20

DALE

LAST VISIT

One Month Later

"DALE, you know the main purpose for today's visit," Dr. Lea prompted. She had already completed his assessments, taking both his history and conducting her examinations, as she did on every visit. Just as before, there were no changes. Dr. Lea didn't leave out her usual string of questions, considering that from one visit to the next there could be changes—and that possibility was true of this visit as well, despite the expected plan. For her, diligence and attention to detail were the keys to excellence.

With regard to her examination, she had taken his vital signs and examined his lungs, heart, and the rest of the cardiovascular system looking for subtle changes that might have indicated anything different from what she had noted on previous exams. Always looking for changes—mainly signs of progression to indicate worsening—she had thoroughly checked him over. For all practical purposes he was stable even with advanced disease. His primary care and specialist physicians were capable of keeping track of him at this point without the active involvement of the palliative care team.

These signs were positive, but Dr, Lea recognized that good news is not always well accepted by the patient and family, since the added attention would no longer be present if the patient were discharged from the palliative care service.

For the doctor in this situation, there is a mild, nagging concern about whether it's actually the right time to discharge the patient: *What if he suddenly deteriorates after being discharged from our care?* This scenario always poses a dilemma, but clinical discernment upon review of the facts, along with an extended course of observation combined with the physician's prior experience, provides assurance of the proper decision. The equation goes something like this: review of the facts plus extended observation plus experience equal physician discernment. All of these factors add up for the physician to confidence that the appropriate decision has been reached. All that was left now was for Dr. Lea to communicate the explanation with the patient.

"Yes, doc. I'm ready. It's good news in a way, isn't it?"

"Right you are! *is* good news. You're doing well enough, and we've accomplished our goals with you, which are really making sure *your* goals are met. Your medical condition is relatively stable. Yes, your lungs are seriously weakened, but there are no signs of change over a number of months, no change in your medical regimen, and you will be fine under the excellent care and attention of your primary care and lung specialist physicians. Are you good with that?"

"Sure. But you're sure it's going to be good news? I mean, on this last visit and all, I'd like to end on good news. You know what I mean?"

"He's stalling," Hannah called out from the kitchen.

"Now, what gave you . . ." Dale started to reply to Hannah. Abruptly, however, at that very moment the front door opened, and the wind blew it out of the hand of the person opening it. The curtain blew out suddenly, striking Dr. Lea. She startled, heart thumping, and quickly turned toward the door to see a man standing there—a stranger, though he looked somehow familiar.

"Am I too late?" he blurted out. Dr. Lea noticed that she was the only one in the room alarmed.

"Aaron, come on in. You're here for the good part. This is Dr. Lea, my PC doctor. She took over for Dr. Dryden," Dale explained.

"Excuse me, Dr. Lea. I'm sorry for interrupting your visit with Dad," Aaron replied.

"Oh, that's fine. I just wasn't expecting anyone else. Nice to have a chance to meet you, and glad you could make it. I'll let you settle in before I proceed."

"He's all set. Keep going, doc," Dale invited her, turning toward the kitchen from his chair. "Might as well join us, too, Hannah. You don't want to miss the fireworks!"

"Fireworks?" Dr. Lea reacted, still slightly unnerved by the unexpected entrance.

"That's just a family thing," Aaron explained. "Never mind him. He always used to say that when something was important."

"Oh, I see. Let me see—where was I?" Dr. Lea asked aloud, mostly of herself.

"Anyone else, Dale? My big punch line is coming, and I don't want anyone else to miss it."

"Doc, you're getting ready to sign off my case, and you're just getting warmed up to fit into the family. Too bad." They all laughed. "You were just getting to know us." Dale winked to his family, and another ripple of laughter ensued.

"Did you hear the one about . . ." Aaron stopped mid-sentence as Dale held up his hand.

"Okay, okay. Now, let's not get out of hand. Doc's got some important words to say to me." Dale, suddenly more serious, was setting a different tone. "Go ahead, doc."

"Thanks, Dale. I enjoy the family bantering back and forth . . . but yes, there is more to say.

"Dale, over these months since I've been visiting you, and even back to the time Dr. Dryden was still seeing you, your advanced lung condition, the COPD, has certainly limited you, and a complex regimen to manage your condition and symptoms has been in place. Over this whole time you've remained stable. You have symptoms, yes, but you're stable. I don't foresee your condition changing dramatically over the next months or even over a longer time period. Before I came today I reviewed our records of your visits and the medications and respiratory regimen you've been on. I'm pleased with how you're doing.

"Recently you've made some drastic changes—or should I say dramatic changes to fit into today's bantering?" She smiled with this comment, and Dale politely smiled back.

"The not smoking is making a big impact on you. Your lungs have long been damaged, and instead of saying 'So what—who cares?' and keeping on smoking, thinking it's too late to make a difference, you've made the much harder choice to quit. This makes your weakened lungs better able to try to do their job. That's an accomplishment, unfortunately, that I don't see very often. See, you keep surprising me."

"That I like to do—surprise you. Aaron's a chip off the ol' block, and he surprised you today too. My stalling helped." Dale slapped his knee hard. Aaron was about to say something, but Dale abruptly held up his hand again and nodded to Dr. Lea.

"Indeed, he did," she concurred. "So, that brings me to the next part about how you're functioning. By this I mean how you're getting along, what you're able to do or not do, and how this is changing over time. This, for me as the physician in charge, is the most important piece to help me look a little way into the future for this decision I need to make—along with you, of course. My experience in the past with similar cases helps too.

"As I said, I believe you're relatively stable. Yes, some unexpected sudden episodes could occur, but they haven't over all these months or more, so why should I expect them now? We haven't had to change anything in the treatment or management of your condition and symptoms. All good with that?"

"Yes," Dale replied. Aaron and Hannah both nodded.

"We also had a major accomplishment with getting your goals of care discussion documented into your finalized advance directive. Signed, sealed, and delivered. That's actually huge! And I congratulate you, Dale. You too, Aaron. Both of you sat down and talked over these important issues and made concrete choices that are central to your planning for the future."

"Dad told me that would be a big help to him and to me. He told me he would have peace spelling out what he wanted for himself for care when he gets really bad. That gives me— no, us—peace too. We worry about those kinds of decisions. Don't we, Hannah?" Dr. Lea gazed at Hannah for her reaction.

"Right, that gives me peace too." Hannah agreed.

"See, Dad." Aaron hesitated, biting his lower lip before continuing, "You worried about being a bad example and that you aren't able to lead us as a father, but you're doing exactly that right now. You're setting a fantastic example of how to plan—not run from the reality of what's happening to you. You know, bury your head in the sand, like you said. It's time to face the reality of what you have and make the most of the time, knowing you're not checking out any time soon. That's being the man of the house, the father figure you wanted to be . . . and you're doing it at the most important time. We can't change what has happened in the past, but we can choose to make the days ahead better. For that I thank you."

"Tissues, anyone?" Hannah offered as she passed them around.

"I couldn't have said it any better. Thanks, Aaron. Glad you're here." Dr. Lea told him.

"All the appropriate communication with your primary care doctor and lung specialist has been done by now. There should be no hiccups in the process of handing things back over.

"I've enjoyed the time meeting and taking care you, Dale. All the best to you." Dr. Lea stood and proffered her hand.

"Thanks, doc. Can't say much else, but you hung in there with me when I wasn't the best—and look at what you've done for me. Can't thank you enough."

"That's enough for me. You're welcome," Dr. Lea replied warmly. Dale signed the requisite paperwork for discharge.

"I'll see you sometime." She felt the need to say something right then, as she was leaving, but wasn't sure this was it.

"For sure, doc." He winked and smiled.

It was quiet in the room as Dr. Lea packed up and exited the home. It was noticeably less windy as she made her way through the door and down the front steps toward her car in the driveway. The sun peeked out from a blue patch of sky behind the billowing gray clouds just at that moment, brightening the yellow and red maple leaves on her car.

21

PEARL

HOSPITAL FOLLOW UP – PAIN AND MORE

Two Weeks Later

PEARL made it to the office on time. She was moving more slowly but remained on her own.

"Pearl, it's so good to see you at the office instead of the hospital. How're you doing?"

"Better, doctor—definitely getting better."

"Again, you've proven how tough you are."

"It's the only way I know; it's my Irish in me." Dr. Lea smiled.

"How's your pain?"

"Yes, well, I'm so glad to have pain medicine. Your office staff told me to tell you I'm using about four breakthrough doses a day and taking the long-acting morphine as you prescribed it last time. Taking my bowel regimen—no problem. The nausea persists, but it's usually milder. I'm taking an ondansetron usually at least once a day. Not eating as much, though. And before you ask, yes, I'm tired."

"Pearl, you gave me a good, rounded report. Your breakthrough dosing is just on the borderline of increasing your long-acting dose. Let's watch you closely and see if your pain or pain medicine use changes. I want to talk to you about something else too. Is that okay?"

"Yes, of course. What is it?" Pearl asked, trying to sit a little straighter.

"Well, I'm concerned about your overall condition and the changes we're seeing with you."

Pearl interrupted, "Doctor, I know what you mean, I think. I want to hear what you have to say."

"Thanks, Pearl. I want you to think about something as we look back over the recent weeks—maybe even the last few months. Your CML seems to be on the verge of progressing to a stage we call transformation."

Pearl replied, "I've heard that word before from Dr. Ludlow. He told me it was coming at my last visit with him. The CAT scans at that time showed some changes that weren't so good. I forget now if it was noticed before or after our last office visit, but anyway, he said it was time to stop the Tykitrol, that in all good conscience he couldn't agree to my taking it anymore. I thought about it then, and I agreed with him. I've stopped it, and I'm not going to restart. I probably should have stopped long ago—but, well, you know the rest of the story: I won't go on and repeat my whole thought process about it.

"Besides, Erin has wanted me to stop it. So has Patrick, I guess," Pearl added.

"I'm glad and relieved you made this decision, and it brings me to my next point. As you're aware, when your CML transforms to AML—as we just discussed, this might be happening in the coming weeks—your time is going to be . . . shorter."

"I understand what you're saying. My life is going to be much shorter than we thought a few weeks or so ago."

"That's right. How do you feel about that . . . now that

we're talking about it?" *Pearl is talking so matter-of-factly. She's handling this better than I am.*

"Dr. Lea, I'm ready. We had that talk weeks ago, and when it came time I accepted it." Pearl paused before continuing, "I want to thank you and the rest of your palliative care crew. I wouldn't have been prepared for all this without you. Besides taking care of my pain and so forth. I want you to know that. You're young and have a long career ahead of you taking care of us people with what you call 'advanced serious illness.' You've learned a lot just over the time you've taken care of me. I've been concerned about you, as I've been seeing myself getting weaker, more tired, doing less, and having more pain.

"Maybe that's why I put on a front sometimes, I think. I tell myself it's for my benefit, but I'm not so sure; it might be more for you. I don't know." She stopped and wiped her eyes with a tissue. "I'm blubbering on here. Can't you say something to help me stop?" Pearl grinned but looked with an almost pleading expression into Dr. Lea's eyes.

"I can do that. I appreciate all you said to me. I've been reminded more than once of my mom during your time in my care. And what I saw her go through—I don't want you to do the same thing. This has been harder for me than I expected. Speaking as a physician, I don't believe I've compromised any integrity in terms of that feeling interfering with my profes-sional decision-making for you . . . at all." They both paused in their conversational exchange.

Dr. Lea continued, "Next, I want to talk with Dr. Ludlow and your primary doctor about referring you to hospice. What are your thoughts about that?"

"Well, let me think about that . . . only because I have an idea in mind. I want to go on a trip with Erin and Patrick and their families. Not far, and not a complicated trip to arrange, but the sooner the better. When I get back we'll do it."

"Pearl, if it's not too far the hospice can arrange a travel contract for where you're going. That way you can still be in hospice care and have access to help if needed."

"But not where I want to go. We have a resort cabin on a small lake three or four hours away from here. It's remote without good access to internet and cell towers." *There she goes, tapping her cheek again.*

"I see. That would be difficult logistically. All right, though, as long as you contact us right away when you return so we can get the hospice referral started. When you know the dates you'll be leaving and returning, then call my office and let us know. It should be less than three weeks from now, though, . . . please. Okay?"

"Yes, Dr. Lea, for sure."

Hugs. Dr. Lea noted Pearl's frailty—her ribs were more prominent due to weight loss— as well as a mild wince.

"You're sure your pain is adequately controlled? You've got to tell me."

"Yes, it is. Really."

"With Erin not here, you'll speak to her about all this?"

"I'll talk to her today. And Dr. Ludlow too."

Dr. Lea walked her to the front desk area of the clinic. Hugs again.

22

PALLIATIVE CARE vs. HOSPICE

PALLIATIVE CARE SUMMARY – 5

Misconceptions and Miscellaneous

Palliative care is easily misunderstood for several reasons.

Many people confuse it with hospice care or think of it as a service that is needed before going into hospice, like a pre-hospice service. Let's talk more about the confusion and help explain how palliative care is different from hospice. It started in hospice care in the United States, but a diagram of the current systems looks like this.

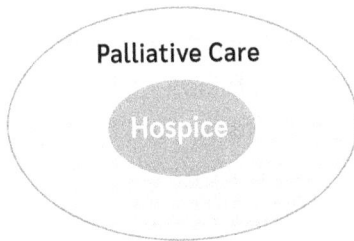

Palliative Care

Hospice

Hospice is a part of palliative care, a specific, or specialized, type of palliative medicine. Hospice is subject to more rules and is more restrictive. To qualify for hospice services a patient must be expected to live only six months or less. That is not true for palliative care, which can be provided alongside aggressive treatments for the underlying disease. Whereas hospice care is intended for the last six months of life, palliative care can be given at any time during a serious illness.

In our two patient stories two different scenarios are portrayed. Dale had a chronic, long-lasting disease but was not on a trajectory toward immediate hospice, whereas Pearl was in palliative care perhaps a little longer than she could have been before being referred to hospice; that referral possibly shortened her PC time, but all along the decline had been unavoidable.

Note also that Pearl had had the serious illness for longer than she received palliative care, making it seem as if her palliative care was for a shorter time. She could actually have benefited from palliative care earlier on if the referral had happened sooner. The reality is that Pearl was in palliative care for an extended time, starting well before the hospice guideline of six months or less. Both patients received specialized palliative care for treatment of symptoms and discussions of goals and planning—key features to make end-of-life care as good as it can be.

Palliative care and hospice use similar language, which can sometimes cause confusion. Using terms like "battle" and "fight" is meant to be helpful when talking about serious diseases, especially cancer. However, this language can cause distress for people with advanced conditions that will likely worsen, such as some types of cancer.

I don't want to take away hope from patients during their treatment, but it's important to have realistic plans based on good medical knowledge, expert opinions, and test results. When treatments for these conditions stop working, it can seem as if the medical staff is out of options and the patient is no longer able to keep fighting. But no one wants to be seen as a quitter, and there will still be plenty to do for the patient (and family) during hospice care.

That's why palliative care physicians and nurses discourage the use of those terms. Let me explain further. Think of the progression from palliative to hospice care as being like filling out a planner. Instead of saying "Don't be a quitter," the providers anywhere along the trajectory can encourage, "So glad you planned ahead." This ensures that the patient has the agency and buy-in ability. The more helpful language on the part of the care providers assures the patient that "your choice is your choice" and that it's "your idea" when to stop treatment. That's why I think of palliative care not as giving up but as making sure.

The thoughtful advance planning can make certain the patent receives the treatment they want—and not the treatment they don't want. It's not about turning the end of every serious illness into a sad story. Rather, it is balancing out the pluses and the minuses, knowing the individual's limits, and being satisfied with the decisions.

This approach helps not only the person who is doing the deciding (whether the patient or a designated decision-maker) but also the important people around them who care about them the most. It lessens the burden, freeing the patient and loved ones from feeling forced to dwell on these difficult and sensitive issues and allowing them to move on in peace and focus on other things in life. Making plans to live one's best with the time the patient still has improves their quality of life.

Fortunately, talking about these important aspects of advanced serious illness doesn't make the possible exigencies happen. For example, talking about CPR doesn't mean the person's heart will stop right away. It does, however, prepare the patient and others around them ahead of time for when decisions will need to be made. This is what I mean by "making sure."

Although palliative care teams talk with patients and families about issues such as CPR, in many situations the topic of discussion does not become an active concern, as the advanced medical condition stabilizes or improves, and there is no immediate need to change direction in treatments and goals or to "call in hospice."

Planning does not necessarily lead to change in the near future, but change, whenever it might be needed, benefits from planning. Palliative care can help the patient and family explore their goals, identify them, pursue them, and reach them. Now, that's quality-of-life planning that is useful and beneficial.

Many palliative care patients, and medical professionals for their part, have a false sense of life expectancy and therefore delay in beginning hospice care. Palliative care usually, but not always, assists in this area. Even with Pearl's considerable palliative care involvement, there was a noticeable delay in terms of the eventual hospice referral. Varying factors play a role in the hospice decision. I explored this thoroughly in the companion book *Hope in Hospice* in the Embrace the Time Series. I explain there how fears and barriers can be addressed to help those involved consider the choice of hospice care earlier.

23

PEARL

IT'S TIME

Thirteen Days Later

"PEARL, you didn't make it the three weeks." Dr. Lea went right into the issue as she entered the clinic exam room.

"Yes, I tried, but the pain got too strong, and the break-through doses haven't been working like they did for the last several days. I had hoped in the past the pain came from something I'd done out in the yard or lifting groceries or vacuuming. Then it would get better if I rested, but that isn't the case anymore. The pain is getting stronger, no doubt. There's a little more burning, and it stays that way. I called Dr. Ludlow, and I'll see him later this afternoon at his office."

"Good—glad you made that appointment too. We need to adjust your long-acting and probably your short-acting doses to make you more comfortable. We can add another medicine to help with the nerve type of pain you're experiencing. It's not a pain medicine per se, but what we call an adjuvant medicine; it helps the pain medicine work better, or the combination of adding it allows for better pain control.

"Also, about your last CT of the abdomen and chest, there is disease progression. It's in the area that makes sense of the worsening pain and the new features that sound like a neuropathic component. I think adding a steroid pill might help. I know you're diabetic, but you're not on any treatment for it, so we'll watch that because steroids can worsen your blood sugar control."

"Okay, Dr. Lea. I'm fine with your plan for the pain medicine and the added steroids. Also, I've had some more nausea. The medicine Dr. Ludlow gave me months or more ago, ondansetron, helped, and your staff gave me a refill on it."

"Good idea. Just check the expiration date on the bottle and be sure it's the newest one we called in for you. If you get heartburn symptoms, let us know that too. The steroids can increase stomach acid and worsen or start heartburn; we call that dyspepsia or reflux."

"You've got a word for everything, doctor." *Smiles.*

"So, your pain became greater, more like a seven or higher? And you said in the same areas—and mild burning with it too?"

"Yes, that's right."

"Let me check you over now." This time the exam results were substantially different. The fullness in the left upper quadrant of the abdomen had a greater degree of fullness, and Dr. Lea felt a larger mass there; Pearl could feel the difference from the exam too. *Splenomegaly made her wince; she never did that before.*

The heart tones were regular, with no murmur or rubs, and the lung sounds, though coarse, were not out of the ordinary for this patient. The right upper quadrant, however, was tender. *This is new. Questionable jaundice on her skin? And her bruising is worse.*

Dr. Lea looked at Pearl's eyes, specifically at the white sclera portions as she gently pulled down the lower eyelids to see if they were at least mildly yellow from jaundice. While examining the head and neck area, Dr. Lea noted that the lymph node on the side of Pearl's neck was larger and that two smaller ones were now present.

"I'm quite concerned, Pearl. There are certain changes on your exam that make me suspect there is disease progression toward the AML transformation. Any gum bleeding or nose bleeds?" At this point Dr. Lea sat back down on her chair but pulled up closer to Pearl so their eyes met at the same level. Pearl closed her eyes as she nodded a yes to the question. Dr. Lea reached for a tissue as small tears formed in the corner of each eye. She gave one to Pearl too.

Pearl took a deep breath, paused, seemed to gather herself, and announced, "Dr. Lea, I think this means you'll get to have only one of my custard birthday pies."

Dr. Lea smiled and dabbed her eyes. "Maybe only the one with you, but I believe I'll have many more, thanks to you. I can still celebrate your birthday even when . . ."

"Indeed, you can!" Pearl picked up the conversational thread quickly. "Grand idea, indeed!" She smiled perhaps her biggest smile ever.

"How was your cabin trip?" Dr. Lea asked while dabbing.

"Oh, we went—not as quickly as I wanted, and we were there for only three days when I had to get back because of all this going on with me. It was worth it, though. Our family had a good time together. The grands had fun in the water and swimming and canoeing with a little bit of fishing. I stayed on shore and watched it all. I had good conversations with Erin and Patrick and spoke with each grandchild one-on-one. It was special to me. I got to tell them I love them and that a part of me will always be with them, right there in their heart."

She made a pointing gesture toward her heart. "I think they got it."

"That sounds like meaningful conversations. You're finishing well. Any questions, Pearl?"

"None. The main focus of the hospice care will be to keep me comfortable and help my family care for me?"

"Yes, Pearl, that's exactly right. All the focus will be on your level of comfort. Tests won't be necessary any longer, since we aren't going to treat the lab numbers or test results but only how you're doing. Are you still okay with that?"

"Yes. What about blood transfusions?"

"In hospice care only if they make a difference, but they can be arranged if they make sense for how you're doing. You'll need to speak with your hospice team. You'll meet a dedicated nurse, called a case manager, and you'll have a social worker assigned as well. They'll be there to help you and your family—that's all.

"The hospice doctors I know personally, and they're top notch; I would trust them with my own family if needed. I will speak with them about your case. Please ask them anything, even the hard questions. They're there for you. As your condition changes the benefits of transfusion become less and less. I'll leave it to their expert knowledge and experience to handle your care and answer your question about transfusions; they'll help you make decisions that are informed and beneficial. Remember, you're in control; no one is taking that away from you. What's important to you will be important to them—count on it.

"Everything related to the hospice condition is completely covered by your insurance. There are no copays for that, no out-of-pocket costs, so don't worry about that, either." Dr. Lea paused here. Pearl sat still, impassive.

"You're fine with me calling the hospice team today to get you seen at your home by the admission nurse? The sooner the better, so we can focus more intensely on getting you more comfortable and getting the added help for you and your family."

Two thumbs up from Pearl.

And a longer hug this time.

24

PEARL

HOSPICE AT HOME

Ten Days Later

"PEARL, thanks for letting me come by today," Dr. Lea announced as she sat at the kitchen table.

"Of course, Dr. Lea. Sorry there's no custard pie for you," Pearl quipped.

Dr. Lea leaned over, picked up a box, and placed it on the table. "Oh, but Pearl, you're in for a big surprise! Here's my version of your custard pie recipe."

"What?! You brought a custard pie? Why, I can't believe it! It looks perfect." Pearl beamed at the sight of the pie.

"Well, the edges didn't turn out quite like yours, but hopefully it tastes close to yours."

"I'm sure it will. We'll see how the bottom crust is when we serve it out, but it looks so far like it won't be soggy. The custard doesn't look gritty or curdled—that's a good sign and what I always look for before I cut into it. The edges aren't shrunken—well, maybe slightly—so you must have let the crust relax before you baked it. Good job, that's a common mistake by beginners. Did the center wobble slightly when you took it out of the oven? I always look for that too."

"Well, I can't recall exactly, but I made it just as your directions say. I took my time—made sure I wasn't on call, so no interruptions."

"Dr. Lea, it looks perfect. Let's eat while it's still chilled. Erin, can you get the small plates and forks out for us? Let's have a slice. I happen to have tea already made, so I must have known somehow, don't you think?"

"For sure, Pearl. You must have," Dr. Lea agreed. *She's paler and looks a little winded. I see some bruises on her skin at the edge of her sleeve. Maybe she needs some oxygen.*

Pearl cut the pie and served it while Erin poured the tea. "The custard is just the right consistency. It's perfect, doctor."

"Well, here's the first bite," Pearl noted as she placed the fork into her mouth and smoothly savored the proper silky texture and the rich, creamy, and gently spiced flavors. "Oh, it's scrumptious, Dr. Lea. I would never have known it was your first custard pie. Very good for a first timer. Congratulations. Eat, eat," Pearl invited Dr. Lea and Erin.

"I wanted to wait and hear what you said about the first bite of the pie. Thanks. Your recipe. And you were inspiring me to try to bake one. I thought that, since I was coming over, I'd bring one to celebrate."

"Celebrate what? It's not my birthday, and I'm in hospice care at home. Is that worth celebrating?"

"Mother . . ." Erin began to say in a slightly chastening tone.

"Why, that's no bother to me," Dr. Lea enthused. "I think we can celebrate that you can still eat custard pie; that it looks like I successfully made my first pie, under your direction; and that you're feeling well enough to be up and around, dressed, and taking guests. From what I've heard you're doing better than expected. So, you're living life and not letting the disease take over and drag you down. With advanced CML transformation into AML, that's something to celebrate." Dr. Lea held up her forkful of custard pie with her right and her cup of tea with her left hand.

"You're right," Pearl responded immediately, and with that she held up her tea to the cheers.

"I've heard from the hospice doctor who visited that you had a good conversation and that he thought he'd answered your questions. He also said you asked about the transfusions. I heard you'd had one set up but canceled it. Why?"

"Truthfully, the last transfusion didn't help me feel much better at all, so I thought it wasn't worth it."

"You made the right call, then. They do come with risks. So, I'm glad you made that choice if they aren't helpful. Everything else going okay?"

"Yes. The pain is much better with the medications you started; I still feel it, but only at a level of two or three. We had a nice visit—glad I got to see him."

"Good. I won't check you over today, since you had a recent visit from the hospice doctor."

"Yes, they poked and prodded plenty. Lots of questions. But he's very good and thorough. Since you recommended him, I trust him right away." Setting down her fork, Pearl changed the subject: "I think I want to go lie down. I'm tired. Erin, can you put the rest of my custard pie piece in the refrigerator, please?" Dr. Lea helped Pearl to the recliner chair.

"I'd do all this myself," Pearl whispered so Erin wouldn't hear in the kitchen, "but I need the help, and she's been good about it. Patrick has been over to give her a break too. It's all going well. I know things are changing."

"Is your faith helping you?"

"Very much so. I pray all the time, and I'm waiting, waiting for the Lord. And surprisingly, I find myself . . . " Pearl slowed and paused. "I find myself not actually being down but almost joyful. This is unexpected, but my faith has never meant as much to me as now. I have peace. I think I'll see Jesus soon."

Still whispering, Pearl continued, "I've noticed more bleeding of my gums and other places too. I don't complain about it and try to clean it up, but I know it probably won't be long that I can still do it. I think that's what you told me—or maybe it was another doctor—that the worsening of the bleeding gums is a late sign. Right? Was that you who said that to me, Dr. Lea?"

"It probably was. Pearl, you look a little winded; you could use some oxygen with your lower blood count. You'll feel better and maybe less tired. It'll help you get around a little better too."

"I have it in the bedroom. I haven't used it yet. If you think it's a good idea, I'll do it."

Pearl reclined more, and within minutes she was sleeping.

Dr. Lea and Erin finished their slices of pie, and Dr. Lea left with the rest, at Erin's insistence.

But Dr. Lea knew. She embraced the time.

25

PEARL

"BE JOYFUL IN HOPE, PATIENT IN AFFLICTION,
FAITHFUL IN PRAYER." ROMANS 12:12

Seventeen Days Later

"DALE, Aaron, Hannah! Is that you? I am so . . ."

"I know, Doc. Don't say it—I'll say it for you: 'I'm so surprised!'" Dale said in his best mimic of Dr. Lea.

"Exactly! What are you doing here?" Dr. Lea asked. She looked around at the formal room of people, some clustered and talking in hushed voices around Erin and Patrick, others sitting on a sofa and crying by themselves, and still others engaged in conversation and laughing softly at an occasional remark. The full continuum of human emotion was on display, not surprising in light of the fact that the deceased had been cherished and that an abundance of fond remembrances were being felt and shared.

Dale explained, "Well, Pearl is my great-aunt. Shocking, isn't it?"

"I can't get over it. I didn't see you through the service, not until now. With your new teeth, your trimmed hair and beard, you look so different."

"It's all good. Glad to run into you, doc. I can't tell you enough how grateful I am for you and the PC team. Without you it could have been me on the receiving end of this service we're at, not my Aunt Pearl. You guys made all the difference. Can't thank you enough for how your team and now the hospice team helped."

"We're just doing our job, caring for you in more ways than one, I guess you could say," Dr. Lea acknowledged.

"Heard you make a mean custard pie."

"How'd you know about that?"

"Well, two days after your visit with Aunt Pearl we went to see her. Heard she was doing bad."

Dr. Lea reminded him, "You told me there was no one else when we had one of our last visits. Why didn't you mention your Aunt Pearl?"

"We weren't on speaking terms yet. And your question was, 'Are you expecting anyone else today?' The truth at that time was no. I didn't expect Aunt Pearl would be there. So, I didn't lie to you, Doc. I wouldn't do that.

"She called me the day after you were there and wanted to see me. She sounded pretty weak over the phone. So, I showed— I mean, *we* showed up the next day. The pie was gone by then, but we heard all about it.

"We cleared the air between us and made things right before she passed. It was her doing, but I feel better about it. She said it was a renewing of her faith that made her want to reconcile. That's what she called it.

"We were close at one time. Mostly back in my music days, but something happened—it's hard to remember what it was all about now, but it is what it is. All is good. She died in peace, doc. Aunt Pearl, she did it right. She lived her life right up to the end. There was no one else like her, eh doc?" Dale finished.

"She is special, that's for sure. *For me, she's the second most special.* Dr. Lea touched a delicate simple gold ring on a matching delicate gold chain necklace.

I've embraced the time, twice.

AFTERWORD

CONTAINED in this book are two patient examples from an endless variety of palliative care patient stories—as many as there are people with advanced serious illnesses. In a single book it would be impossible, of course, to touch on every patient's experience or diagnosis. Still, the principles of palliative care are evident through these records of individual patient/clinician visits.

One example offered in the book is that of a patient who eventually entered hospice care following an extensive palliative care experience. You can see throughout how palliative care helped in decision-making through discussion about patient goals involving family, advance care planning, and attentive symptom management. The other case covered in the book is that a patient whose trajectory of illness improved while in palliative care, who did not need hospice care, and who was able to return to his primary care and specialist physicians for ongoing stable symptom management from advanced serious illness.

The interspersed factual chapters were meant to expound on related material that is important but not directly connected to the stories of the patients. I hope they did not interfere with the flow of the patients' stories but helped with understanding the big picture as the stories moved along. Still other material related to understanding palliative care but not directly related to the patient stories is placed in the following Appendix.

Altogether, the collection of stories chronicling the patients' experiences with advanced serious illnesses, along with the factual information presented collectively, shows how with palliative care these patients were able to live more . . . "More" in this context does not necessarily equate to longer. Think of "more" as in living more fully and, in that sense, living better— better in terms of quality of life, though not necessarily in quantity or length.

More of life, living with a better quality of life. That's not easy to achieve; in fact, it takes courage to live each day when faced with serious illness. So, why not consider palliative care to enable "more" of what the patient wants with less struggle from the symptoms and burden of disease, illness, condition, or treatment? This doesn't at all mean giving up on treatment, life, or oneself.

It's more about making sure. If you are the patient, it's making sure that your care and treatment are what you want to match your goals, wishes, and desires for the way you want to be treated and cared for—for how you want to live. You are in control, or someone you trust is making decisions for you according to the road map you created with your advance directive.

This gives you relief from a load of burden, suffering, and stress (whether physical, social, mental, emotional, or spiritual), so you can concentrate on what is important to you; it gives you renewed vigor for focus. This affords fulfilling peace and hope that are meaningful and satisfying. Give yourself the best chance for this with an engaged, expert, caring, and guiding palliative care team.

APPENDIX

Brief History

PALLIATIVE CARE is a specialty recognized by physician groups, hospitals, insurance companies, Medicaid, and Medicare. You might have to pay copays or follow certain rules about your own or your loved one's care. There are programs in hospitals, in outpatient clinics, embedded in cancer centers, in dialysis centers, and in skilled nursing facilities. Many times this care can also occur in patients' homes.

Modern palliative care entered the picture somewhat alongside hospice care, the latter of which had its beginnings in the UK with Dr. Cicely Saunders. However, the contemporary concept of palliative care, with its unique principles and approach to the care of non-terminal but serious illness, rose to the fore in the 1960s. Balfour Mount, a medical doctor, is recognized as the founder of palliative care in North America. He played a key role in the development, teaching, and expansion of the concept to other countries in the following decades. Dr. Mount passed away in 2025.

More on Palliative Care confusion with Hospice

Many people think that palliative care is either the same as hospice care or that it's a way for others to push them into hospice. That is almost never the case, although there are uncommon exceptions. It is true that palliative care is sometimes considered a bridge to hospice care when the patient, though not ready for hospice, is in an obvious hospice-eligible situation for those with very advanced diseases who are doing very poorly. Another scenario is when the individual might need assistance for symptom treatment while continuing (or exploring) aggressive treatment for a time; regular support through close, expert clinical follow up from a palliative care team can help in this situation.

Below is a table comparing palliative care with hospice care. The most important difference is that hospice requires that the patient has been given a six-months-or-less prognosis (this is what is meant by being "terminal") for eligibility, whereas palliative care can be provided for patients with an advanced serious illness at any time throughout their illness.

Hospice may restrict certain procedures or medications not intended strictly for comfort, since comfort is the intention of hospice care—not trying to cure or improve the condition to prolong life, as the rest of the medical field is trying to do. These restrictions do not exist for palliative care, which provides care alongside the treatments for the underlying disease from the primary care or specialty care services. For additional information on hospice, see the companion volume of *Hope in Hospice*.

	PALLIATIVE CARE	HOSPICE
Patient Eligibility for the Care	Anyone with serious illness, at any time during the course of illness	*Terminal* prognosis of less than 6 months *required*
Real-Time Care with Cure Care	Yes	No
Who Pays	Medicare, Medicaid, insurance	Medicare, Medicaid, insurance

	Medicare Part B	Medicare Part A
Medicare Billing Category	Medicare Part B	Medicare Part A
Who Provides	Consultant, team	Hospice team always
Setting of Care	Any location	Nearly any
Treatment Restrictions	None	Probably, since comfort care only
Timing during the Course of Serious Illness	Any	End-of-life: 6 months prognosis required
Proven to Reduce Costs	Yes	Yes

Palliative care has a unique history among medical specialties, which makes it difficult to see the differences between it and hospice care. Hospice care, the more specialized form, started before the broader field of palliative care, whereas other areas of medical specialties have developed differently.

As a contrasting example, cardiology started first, before its subspecialties like interventional, electrophysiology, structural, and pediatric cardiology. After the general specialty core focus was established, over time and through research it became clear that the depth and amount of information and experience had grown, leading to more specialized knowledge and, eventually, to better specialized care. Dedicated doctors and teams focus only on subspecialized levels of care to become more highly skilled at them, thereby creating a new subspecialty.

There is an interesting point to consider about communication when a patient doesn't want palliative care. During those times people in the medical field will often say that "the patient is not ready for palliative care." This statement would not be made of a patient experiencing chest pain and being referred to cardiology for evaluation.

This demonstrates that even many medical professionals misunderstand palliative care, portraying it as a place a patient would want to avoid. There is room on both sides for more education for everyone, as well as better communication between physicians and specialists and between physicians and patients. We must keep focusing on the need for improved communication.

There are additional reasons people confuse the two specialties. One is that the same professionals, including physicians and advanced practice nurses, handle both aspects of patient care. There aren't many other fields like this today. An example of this from the past was that Ear, Nose, and Throat (ENT) doctors also treated eyes; they had originally been called Eyes, Ears, Nose, and Throat (EENT) specialists. As it became clear that eye doctors were most effective when they focused only on eyes, ophthalmology emerged as its own field, separate from ear, nose, and throat medicine.

Another example of two fields that are losing their connection is Hematology and Oncology. Today the training for the two overlaps, but most doctors choose to focus on either blood disorders (benign or malignant diseases) or oncology. In hospice and palliative care training programs, the training throughout is joint. In reality, however, it is becoming more and more separated, especially in larger cities and health systems. However, many clinicians still practice the two together.

Another reason for misunderstanding is that a patient can transition from palliative care to hospice care, or vice versa, which is not usually the case with the other combined specialties mentioned above. This can cause confusion for patients.

More advance directives information
on decision-making

Following are a few important concepts and terms that are often confused, but it is crucial between the two systems to keep their respective meanings separate and to understand how they are used in decision-making. *Competency*, for example, is not the same as *capacity*. Competency is a legal decision made by the court and judges, not an official evaluation and judgment that follows legal rules.

A doctor can determine if a patient has the medical capacity (the ability to do something at a particular moment) to make complex decisions regarding their health and medical care or treatment. From a doctor's point of view, I see capacity as a determination of whether a patient can understand (grasp) what is happening when they learn about their medical condition and the possible results of the choices they will make about it. Think of GRASP as an acronym, as follows:

» **G**et it – Does the patient understand what they are being told medically about themselves?

» **R**eason it – Can the patient think through the implications of a medical decision?

» **A**pply it – Is the patient able to apply what they were told in terms of their values and goals?

» **S**tate it – Can the patient express their understanding and wishes?

» **P**ersistence – When the patient is asked to repeat or explain their choice or understanding, does the decision stick with them, or are there signs of change in their thoughts, reasoning, application, and ability to express ideas?

If a patient cannot grasp information regarding their medical condition sufficiently to make a rational and consistent decision, they lack the capacity to make these decisions. This determination can fluctuate, which can make these situations difficult. The capacity determination can change, but the legal determination of competency is not so easily changed. To be legally competent a person must have the ability (capacity) to think clearly. I know these concepts are confusing, but the distinctions are important to remember.

A person who is deemed incompetent cannot legally create or change an advance directive document. This is another good reason to fill out an advance directive before a crisis occurs.

More pain topics

Chronic pain Chronic pain isn't just pain the patient experiences over a long period of time; the situation is much more complicated than that. Chronic pain may start with an injury or illness. But as the patient heals the pain persists; it feels very real and *is* real. Why does this occur for some people but not for others? What makes it happen, and how does someone make this persistent pain go away? What is known is that the treatment for the pain when it started is not the same as the needed treatment when it becomes chronic. If the same treatment method is used for long-term pain as for short-term pain, this can actually complicate the situation by creating more issues.

When palliative care patients ask me to help with their chronic pain, I have to say no because I don't have the right level of expertise to treat it effectively. Instead, I will work with their primary care doctor and a pain specialist. This way everyone understands what is happening and who is in charge of each part of the program to manage the pain. This ensures that there are no adverse interactions or other problems between the medications prescribed or treatments provided by the different doctors.

Some patients might not like this setup, but that is the way it's usually handled. I explain to the patients that they deserve the best care for what they're going through, so it's important to get the right specialist involved for successful pain treatment. Each palliative care program is independent, and they can organize their services and care for patients in different ways.

Chronic pain is a multifaceted condition that involves deep neurological pathways and includes brain centers that are not affected by other types of pain treated by the palliative care team. That is why patients experiencing this type of pain need a physician and other team member specialists trained specifically in chronic pain management to provide a comprehensive approach to treating it.

Malignant pain Malignant pain is pain that happens due to the effects of cancer on the body. Its management might also include dealing with the way the treatment affects the body and causes pain. The treatments include chemotherapy, immunotherapy, radiation therapy, or cancer surgery. The palliative care team is skilled at understanding these kinds of pain and then creating an effective plan.

Identifying types of pain A patient's palliative care provider will ask how the pain feels and ask the person to rate it. They will also ask when the pain is felt, how it changes, and if there are specific times of day or night when it gets better or worse. Are there specific aspects or qualities of the pain the patient notices, such as aching, sharp, hot, burning, or shooting pain, especially when the patient is moving or engaged in certain activities? What makes the pain better or worse? A patient can experience multiple kinds of pain at the same time, even from the same illness, and the palliative care team will ask about each type to better understand how the pain feels and how it is reacting to the current treatment plan.

Opioid rotations When we change from one opioid to another, we refer to this as opioid rotation. The best times to change the medicine are when the opioid isn't working well, the side effects are too severe to handle, an allergic reaction occurs, or there could be dangerous interactions with other medications. These are all good reasons to try a different pain medicine.

The palliative care provider, whether a physician, nurse practitioner, or physician assistant, has experience in handling these rotations, and there are proven methods for switching safely and effectively between opioids. The patient can help by reporting any side effects from the change and by keeping track of how much prescribed medication they are using. This helps the palliative care team change the dose if needed. It may also indicate that an additional medication is needed.

The new medication might be a stronger opioid than the original pain medicine, especially if the first one is no longer helping. It could also be a different type or class of opioid, since some work better than others for certain kinds of pain, and different people can react differently to strong pain medications.

Soon there will be easy lab tests available to help doctors find the right pain medication for a patient. This is already happening for other types of medication, but the tests are not usually administered outside specialized clinics, advanced care centers, or research facilities. When these tests do become readily available, they will offer much more effective treatment of malignant pain.

Another feature of the rotation is getting the pain better managed with short-acting forms of the pain medicine and then using that amount of opioid to convert to more convenient long-acting forms of it. The extended-release form smooths out the pain control over the course of twenty-four hours, offers better convenience with one to three doses per day, and thereby enhances patient compliance. The short-acting form is still available for any pain between the long-acting doses. This kind of plan is calculated and modified as needed for the best results for the patient.

Adjuvant medicines Add-on medications are called adjuvants. They could be steroids, anti-inflammatories, antidepressants, antiseizure medications, or several other types of specialized medications. Be aware that some of the uses for these medications are considered to be off lab, meaning that the medication is being used for a reason not officially approved by the FDA. This is not at all uncommon. For example, there are many times when a doctor may use an antibiotic for an infection that is not on the official FDA approved list. Physicians have the ability to do this and have been doing so for many years. This discretionary use is actually an important aspect of medicine.

SPECIAL COMMENT ON MARIJUANA/CANNABIS The use of marijuana/cannabis for helping to treat pain is a controversial and complex issue from both a medical and a legal standpoint. It is considered an adjuvant medicine and is neither an opioid nor related to opioids. There is no strong or convincing evidence to support its use for treating pain, and it is not therefore considered a standard recommendation for pain treatment.

In general, adjuvant medicines belong to a group of medicines that help treat pain. Following are some examples by their generic names, though this list is not exhaustive:

Category	Medication
Non-opioid Pain Medicine	Acetaminophen
Anti-inflammatory	Ibuprofen
Anti-inflammatory	Naproxen
Anti-inflammatory	Diclofenac
Common Opioids for Pain	Hydrocodone with acetaminophen
Common Opioids for Pain	Morphine
Common Opioids for Pain	Hydromorphone
Common Opioids for Pain	Fentanyl
Common Opioids for Pain	Oxycodone
Common Opioids for Pain	Methadone
Uncommon Opioids	Buprenorphine
Uncommon Opioids	Codeine
Uncommon Opioids	Tramadol
Other	Marijuana/Cannabis— not recommended
Adjuvant Medication - Steroids	Dexamethasone
Adjuvant Medication - Steroids	Prednisone
Adjuvant Medication - Antidepressants	Amitriptyline
Adjuvant Medication - Antidepressants	Doxepin

Adjuvant Medication - Antidepressants	Duloxetine
Adjuvant Medication - Antidepressants	Nortriptyline
Adjuvant Medication - Antidepressants	Sertraline
Adjuvant Medication - Antidepressants	Venlafaxine
Adjuvant Medication - Antidepressants	Mirtazapine
Adjuvant Medication - Antiseizure (anticonvulsants)	Gabapentin
Adjuvant Medication - Antiseizure (anticonvulsants)	Pregabalin
Adjuvant Medication - Antiseizure (anticonvulsants)	Topiramate
Adjuvant Medication - Other	Ketamine
Adjuvant Medication - Other	Oral rinse or combinations
Adjuvant Medication - Other	Topical compounded creams

Interventional pain techniques As pain worsens, or when it is severe from the start, there are opportunities for interventional pain procedures to help lessen the severity; these are aimed at reducing the need for and the amount of strong pain medicine. It is rare that these procedures are performed by a palliative care practitioner, since mastering the techniques requires years of additional training beyond the baseline specialty of anesthesia or physical medicine and rehabilitation.

The benefit of using the intervention is that raising the dose of the opioid can cause more adverse effects, so it is best to avoid high doses of opioids when possible. The palliative care provider helps assess the need for interventions and refers patients to other interventional pain specialists or primary care providers to help as needed. The interventional services a particular community offers also affect the practicality of such a referral.

Interventional pain management is the term for using procedures to treat pain. These are typically done in a pain clinic with physician specialists. The chosen procedure prevents the nerve from sending pain signals; the focus of the procedure is not on what is causing the pain. Some examples of these procedures are radioablation, which uses heat from electrical current; cryoablation, which uses cold; and chemical ablation, which involves injecting a chemical.

All of these methods destroy the nerve, causing it to stop sending pain signals. Some common terms for these techniques are cautery, ablation, and nerve blocks. Another technique, called nerve stimulation, is a procedure in which an implant device is placed for a chemical reservoir of pain medicine that flows directly to the nerve or a wire that is placed in the body in or near the spine to keep up a steady, small electrical current to block the nerve near the spinal cord.

These procedures are handled very precisely to target only the specific nerve that carries the pain signals, using imaging x-rays, CT scans, or MRI for guidance in placement. Typically this treatment is done on an outpatient basis, meaning that the patient will not need to stay overnight in the hospital. First, test doses are given to confirm that the correct nerve is temporarily blocked for relief. After that a more permanent procedure is performed to provide long-lasting pain relief.

The benefits of these interventions include not only long-lasting pain relief but also the advantage of a reduced need for strong opioid and adjuvant medicines. Sometimes complete response of the pain to these procedures will allow safe and complete withdrawal from the pain medications.

If that is not possible, then at least a significant dose reduction may be an option. That is a very positive thing, since when the patient's pain level is significantly reduced they are spared from side effects of the opioid or other pain medicine, and other possible actions of the opioid or pain medication on the body are eliminated. Another plus is that withdrawal allows the same opioid to work better later on if the pain returns or worsens, because the body will not already be accustomed to its effects.

Specialized pain Specialized types of pain can include neuropathy, mixed pain types, pain when swallowing, mouth pain, and pain from radiation. Palliative care specialists are trained to understand the type of pain a patient is experiencing and to create a treatment plan to safely reduce that pain in a way that works for the patient. A review of these types of pain and possible treatment options has already been provided. This includes using the extra medications mentioned above.

Additional symptoms for palliative care

Nausea/vomiting Nausea and vomiting are very common gastrointestinal symptoms treated by palliative care teams. Medications are very effective at managing these symptoms quickly and are also used for long-term cases of nausea and vomiting. These are especially common in patients with cancer conditions caused either by the disease itself or by the cancer treatments, including chemotherapy and radiation therapy.

The impact of nausea and vomiting extends beyond the gastrointestinal system to include appetite and weight loss and anxiety, especially a particular form of anticipatory nausea and vomiting. This special form is related to the timing of the patient's expectation of cancer treatment; the patient's anxiety is reflected in the symptoms of nausea. Sometimes antinausea medications are used ahead of cancer treatments to prevent the symptoms from happening at all. Coordination with the cancer-treating team is important to successfully treat nausea and vomiting associated with the disease and its treatments.

Constipation Constipation is a very common symptom. It can be caused by the disease, diet, or medications, especially pain medications. The opioid pain medication class so commonly leads to constipation that the experience of every patient needs to be addressed. This is common because the receptor that is acted upon by the pain medicine is in the intestinal tract lining, causing a sluggish motility function of the stomach and intestine.

Constipation doesn't go away over time, as do some of the other side effects, such as nausea and vomiting or drowsiness. It is uncommon, in fact, that someone taking opioids does not need to take medicine to keep their bowels moving regularly and comfortably. The patient taking opioids should make sure their palliative care provider talks to them about constipation and their bowel habits. Some other medicines can lead to the same problem.

There are very common bowel regimens that are effective. If one doesn't work, typically adding another medicine from a different class will work in a different way to provide the desired effect. As a side note, in palliative care it is sometimes not recommended to use only a fiber-based product for managing constipation, as adequate hydration is necessary for it to work effectively. If the patient cannot drink oral liquids in adequate quantity, the fiber product will be ineffective. Also note that there are many home remedies to treat constipation. It is important for the patient to tell the palliative care provider if they are using these to be sure there are no drug interactions or troubling effects.

Diarrhea Diarrhea is much less common but can be a difficult symptom to treat. The medications currently available have been around for a long time, without many newer options available. Diarrhea can be caused by the disease; diet; surgery; medications, including chemotherapy and immunotherapy; and radiation therapy. Additionally, there are times when an infection within the intestine may cause diarrhea. The patient's provider will need to pay close attention to help sort this out.

This issue, when not easily managed, will frequently require referral to a gastrointestinal specialist to help figure it out, using tests, labs, or procedures to assist in diagnosis. If diarrhea is not managed properly it can lead to dehydration and problems with electrolytes, which can sometimes be serious. It is important for the patient to be cautious and inform their provider.

Appetite Appetite management can be difficult, and there are no consistently effective medications available. A term to be aware of is anorexia, meaning loss of appetite. In the context of this discussion it is not related to the anorexia nervosa disorder. There are many home remedies as well. It is important that the patient tell the provider about their home remedies if they are going to prescribe something. Medicines in this category include steroids, cannabinoids, antidepressants, and a few others. For cancer patients appetite loss can be difficult to manage successfully. Sometimes a referral to a nutritionist or dietitian can help.

A separate factor to consider is cancer cachexia. This is a fancy term to describe the condition, which includes severe weight loss, with or without loss of appetite, and a decrease in food and calorie intake. There are clinics that specialize in this disorder, and studies show that a complex internal metabolic process leads to these symptoms. There are currently not many therapeutic options.

Anxiety/depression/insomnia These symptoms are also very common. There are a variety of medications used for label and off-label use to treat these symptoms. The treatments and medications have improved over the past ten or more years, so a good result is likely. Sometimes a combination of medication and referral to behavioral specialists is helpful. Also, there are psychologists in the field known by a variety of terms for their subspecialty. Some of these include behavioral oncology, cancer psychosocial therapy, psycho-oncology, cancer therapists, or cancer counselors.

Fatigue Both primary fatigue from the underlying disease and lack of rest due to disease, treatment, or intervention are troubling for many patients. Review of proper sleep and rest steps is important, as these will take care of most fatigue/sleep-related symptoms. It is also necessary to address the patient's activity level and the addition of exercise to their routine. This does not mean that the patient should be on a marathon training program, but regular, gentle exercise with simple weights and resistance exercises, along with safe walking or biking regularly, can help.

If fatigue persists and is either overwhelming or disruptive of life activities, medication management can be attempted. This is usually done with oral steroids or stimulants, such as those used for treating ADHD. There are steps the doctor will review with the patient to safely consider these medications for the patient's fatigue.

With regard to stimulants, this may include evaluation for contraindicated conditions of anxiety disorders; poorly controlled hypertension; heart disease, including arrythmias; or overactive thyroid conditions. There are multiple conditions for which steroids may not be considered, including diabetes mellitus, severe gastric conditions, recent gastrointestinal bleeding, or the use of anticoagulants like aspirin, warfarin, and direct oral anticoagulants. There are other factors to consider, as well, that the prescribing provider will review with the patient.

Other symptoms, conditions, or topics There are less frequent symptoms that palliative care can also help manage. These include severe sweats or night sweats; excessive airway secretions like mucus; trouble swallowing; and others.

When patients living with serious advanced illnesses face situations in which an intervention could impact their quality of life or extend their life, a palliative care consultation is needed and helpful. This individualized approach will consider the patient's wishes (ideally described in an advance directive) and current medical conditions to help with a decision. For this assessment it's important to work closely with the patient's primary care physician and specialists. The circumstances below are often encountered.

Artificial feeding or tube feeding The decision whether to introduce artificial feeding is complicated and fraught with emotion. I believe that the concept of bridge feeding helps to sort through it. Think of artificial feeding as a bridge that helps the patient reach a destination, just as a road bridge facilitates travel.

If you want to get from one side of a lake, river, or steep valley to the other, a bridge can help you cross without your having to drive around and waste time and miles. It would take much less time and fewer miles to go straight over the hurdle instead of all the way around in a circuitous route to reach the destination. Artificial feeding is like a bridge when the obstacle is preventing the individual from getting the right amount of nutrition and fluids.

This is exactly what happens when an advanced serious illness interferes with the patient's ability to swallow food and fluids. If, despite the risks, the use of artificial feeding helps the patient recover, gain strength, or prevent complications, it makes sense to use it, especially if the swallowing issue is temporary. This would also make sense for a patient without an advanced serious illness facing the same kind of obstacle, likely due to an injury from an accident or a sudden severe illness.

Sometimes bridge feeding can also be a sensible option for a person with a serious illness who is remaining active and managing their life on their own terms. In such a situation artificial feeding will help the patient get over the bridge to allow time for them to heal or improve in order to reach health, their destination. However, when the route over the bridge (the artificial feeding) won't lead to the destination of healing, improvement, or prevention of complications, that course of action is worth reconsidering to see if it aligns with the patient's goals and wishes.

Feeding tubes come with risks because they entail a type of surgery in which an artificial tube is placed into the stomach, either through the mouth or through the abdominal wall. Risks include infection, bleeding, displacement (when something falls out), and problems related to anesthesia, among others.

These conversations are tough to have, and there is no one correct answer that fits all scenarios. But the point at which this kind of intervention might come under consideration is an opportune time to weigh out the specific factors related to the patient's desired quality of life. Sometimes a trial of the feeding tube can be helpful to see how it will affect the patient in the near future.

Conditions in which the discussion of artificial feeding may apply include all types of dementia, strokes, ALS (Lou Gehrig's Disease), and sometimes cancers or cancer treatments that affect swallowing. There are other, less frequent conditions for which this might also apply. The patient, their doctors, and other healthcare professionals can start a palliative care consultation to help with this conversation.

Code status or resuscitation This is another emotionally charged situation, similar in that way to a discussion of artificial feeding. The context of this discussion as it is dealt with throughout this book is the importance of understanding what the patient wants in consideration of their overall health, hopes, and the involvement of the people who matter to them, as well as of the medical teams. You might see the abbreviation DNR or DNAR, which mean the same thing: Do Not Attempt Resuscitation.

Research shows that the chance of a patient with advanced serious illness returning to their previous level of health and functioning—being "successful"—is very low when they undergo resuscitation to restore their heartbeat and breathing. Attempting to revive someone can lead to harmful effects both immediately and later on, and these should be considered when making decisions about resuscitation attempts. Again, no single choice works for every situation, and everyone has the right to choose what is best for themselves. Changes in condition are opportunities for these discussions to happen.

As an example of necessary ongoing discussion between the decision makers and the medical team, early on after a sudden severe illness happens, there may be a time period of unknown length and uncertainty of the patient's long-term outcome. This period of time could be hours or days or a few weeks even. How the patient does during this period may impact further medical care decisions, especially those that surround the patient's resuscitation or code status.

Ventilators or breathing machines and kidney dialysis When a person's lung or kidney function worsens during a serious illness, this is another important time to think about their goals and wishes. This can help decide whether using a breathing machine or starting (or continuing) dialysis is a good option. All of the factors we have talked about earlier apply to these situations too.

In addition, a breathing machine decision is necessary when discussing and deciding about code status, chest compressions or DNAR. This is because without giving adequate oxygen by the ventilator (which requires a tube placed down the throat into the major lung passages) doing the chest compressions that forces the blood around the body in the blood vessels (the circulation) will not deliver oxygen around the body, including very importantly the brain, it will not work as well for best results. So, both parts of resuscitation need to be addressed, the chest compressions for circulation and the breathing part of getting oxygen into the body; the two systems work together.

Other life-prolonging procedures The same basic ideas from the previous discussions apply to many other situations in which planned treatment will affect a patient's overall health and life expectancy. Taking advantage of these opportunities would ordinarily be the right way to respond to them. Expert guidance from a palliative care team can be very important when dealing with complex medical issues that have ethical ramifications.

Conditions and symptoms not managed by palliative care

It is important to understand this group of symptoms and chronic conditions that are outside the specialty of palliative care (several examples are included at the end of this Appendix, but this list is by no means exhaustive). There can be differences among programs, so the list is not necessarily accurate or completely true for every program.

Acute catastrophic injury or illness

It is important to talk about how palliative care (PC) relates to patients in the hospital. While this book does not cover the care and treatment of PC in a hospital setting, in many communities caring for hospitalized patients is the main function of palliative care. This fits into the category I mentioned earlier in the book about not being able to cover all possible scenarios in which PC is suitable for patients.

The idea of having important conversations when dealing with serious illness applies here as well. For the PC provider this means listening carefully, giving full attention, staying focused, and understanding what the patient or their caregivers and family know about their condition and want to learn. It also involves working together with the doctors and medical team to ensure that everyone is on the same page, thereby preventing misunderstandings and mixed messages.

Palliative care also tries to anticipate medical situations ahead of time and give guidance to help prepare for them, should they materialize.

At the heart of this kind of discussion is understanding what the patient wants for their healthcare. Yes, that's right—let's go back to the roadmap of the advance directive. This information is crucial to understanding the direction of care the patient desires, so they can be advised, supported, and enabled to pursue their goals appropriately.

In the setting of life-threatening injury or illness, these discussions happen unexpectedly and urgently and tend to be medically complex, which makes it even more important to have guidance pointed in the direction of the patient's goals.

If the patient hasn't filled out an advance directive and can't make decisions, family members have to take responsibility. The order of priority for responsibility is determined by the location of the medical care. This can be different from state to state, and sometimes there are even differences within counties in the same state. The hospital social worker, palliative care team, and legal adviser will know the requirements and be able to determine the right person.

In this case an undesignated person—at least not formally designated by the patient—will be asked to make the decisions. This person can act on their personal knowledge of the patient's choice, if that was talked about previously. If that information isn't known, the decision-maker usually decides based on what a reasonable person would do or think best for the patient. There are small differences between these two points, as discussed in medical ethics, but in practice they are very similar.

The undesignated decision-maker is responsible for making the final decision. If they refuse to do so, then, based on the hierarchy or order of responsibility established for the hospital, the staff will ask for others to participate in the decision-making. If no one takes responsibility, they will typically look for a professional guardian to make decisions for the patient.

This necessitates going to court, which takes time and usually delays medical care at those decision points while waiting for the court's process to unfold. Once again, having an advance directive prepared and properly activated in such a situation will help ensure that the patient receives timely and proper care.

Examples of complex medical situations with critical issues of care include the following: cardiac resuscitation, do not attempt resuscitation (DNAR), breathing support by ventilator, long-term feeding methods, dialysis for failing kidneys, and possible surgeries. Sometimes the decisions made at the moment will lead to further decision options down the road.

If, for example, a ventilator is used to help someone breathe in an emergency, and they do not start breathing on their own after a few days to a couple of weeks later, a decision will need to be made about surgically inserting a permanent breathing tube; this procedure is called a tracheostomy. Often at the same time the patient will have trouble swallowing, and it may for that reason be necessary to use a feeding tube that is also inserted surgically. This tube is usually known as a PEG tube. Decisions about these choices will once again depend on the patient's wishes and goals, if they are known.

There are no clear right or wrong decisions, but making a choice with the goal of following what the patient wishes is usually the best and clearest approach. If that is not feasible, the determination goes back to deciding in the manner of a reasonable person what is in the patient's best interest. These are difficult situations to be in and to sort through, so getting help from experts is a good idea. The palliative care team is the medical team that helps support the family and the person making the decisions.

In this section we did not go over specific patient cases or examples, but the main ideas remain the same. These scenarios feel more important and urgent because the situation is developing quickly and seriously. If a patient or their loved ones find themselves in this situation, having a palliative care team to support them will help make a difference.

Symptoms not usually managed by pallliative care programs

Chronic Pain
Chronic Headache or Migraines
Nutrition Deficiency
Addiction
Opioid Use Disorder or Other Substance Use Disorders
Seizures
Orthopedic Conditions
Chronic Infections

Chronic medical diagnoses or conditions not usually managed by palliative care

Neurologic Disorders (exception for specific non-neurologic symptoms that might be addressed by Palliative Care)

Multiple Sclerosis
Parkinson's Disease
Alzheimer's Dementia and Other Types
Stroke

The following are examples of chronic illness commonly managed by primary care providers or other specialists prior to late or advanced stages; further diagnostic or therapeutic, condition-specific interventions are managed by the primary and specialty physicians. However, the following list gives an idea of chronic conditions in this category:

Diabetes Mellitus
Hypertension
Arthritis
Heart Disease
COPD/Asthma
Kidney Failure
Rashes and Skin Ulcers or Wounds

NOTES

1. Nichols, Ralph G., PhD, and Stevens, L. A. *Are You Listening: The Science of Improving Your Listening Ability for a Better Understanding of People.* McGraw-Hill. 1957.

2. Cox, C. L. *Patient understanding: How should it be defined and assessed in clinical practice?* J Eval Clin Pract. 2023 Oct;29(7):1127-1134. doi: 10.1111/jep.13882. Epub 2023 Jun 20. PMID: 37338517.

3. 2024 Edition: *Hospice Facts and Figures.* Alexandria, VA: National Alliance for Care at Home.

4. Byock, Ira, MD. *The Four Things That Matter Most: A Book about Living.* New York. Free Press, 2004.

RESOURCES AND REFERENCES

Albom, Mitch. *Tuesdays With Morrie*. London, England. Sphere, 1997.

Harriman, Gerald. *Hope in Hospice*. Grand Rapids. Credo House Publishers, 2025.

Online resources for finding a palliative care program: getpalliativecare.org and PalliativeDoctors.org.

Steinbeck, John. *Grapes of Wrath*. New York. Viking Press, 1939.

ACKNOWLEDGMENTS

To Nancy, my wife, words cannot begin to convey my appreciation for your enduring love and commitment to our lives together. Your dedication to our family and friends remains one of your best qualities, among the many others. You put up with my marathon writing sessions, even another time around on this second book. I couldn't do it without you, ever. Thank you.

To Mike, for your encouragement to improve my writing and understand the writing industry through familiarity with other successful writers. I see that as a genuine push you've given me to be better. Thank you.

To Marie, for your enduring interest, support, and nuggets of suggestion to improve the book. Thank you.

To Barb, for your thorough and vital review of the manuscript and your important and careful suggestions to make it better, clearer, and more correct. Thank you.

To Dr. Caitlin Fulton, for your clinical review and thoughtful input to ensure that I included what needs to be there in just the right way for the reader to get the full view of palliative care. And for doing it despite the great and fulfilling work you yourself are engaged in. Thank you.

To those many others who have asked me about how it's going, encouraged me to keep writing, or given me positive reinforcement and prayed for me throughout the writing and rewriting process. Some of these include our Auntie Jeanne, our small group, our recent friend David, and my friend Jack. Thank you.

A special thanks to our friends Dennis and Naomi, who listened to me talk about the book and did not throw me out of their house or the restaurant booth. Thank you.

Sincere, appreciative thanks to Tim Beals and his staff at Credo House Publishers for their expert review, editing, and design for the book to make it the best it can be for the readers' experience. That is, after all, the goal: to write and publish a book for the reader to gain needed knowledge or answers and to enjoy the experience along the way.

ABOUT THE AUTHOR

Dr. Gerald Harriman is dually board certified in both hospice and palliative medicine and family medicine. He graduated from Michigan State University College of Osteopathic Medicine and has a combined active medical practice of nearly forty years. Besides his family practice he worked for Harbor Hospice in Muskegon, Michigan, as their medical director for over eighteen years. He drew upon all these years of experience to write this book, which is intended to help others not just to learn about palliative care but to gain a glimpse into its workings in providing care for individuals dealing with advanced serious illness.

Dr. Harriman is a distinguished Fellow of the American Academy of Hospice and Palliative Medicine and is recognized for his professional accomplishments in the field. He is a Paul Harris Fellow from the Rotary Foundation and an associate professor at Michigan State University College of Osteopathic Medicine. He was recognized as a Teacher of the Year Award recipient for Hospice and Palliative Medicine in the Trinity (Mercy) Health Grand Rapids fellowship program.

Dr. Harriman was born and raised in Grand Rapids, Michigan, and has practiced medicine throughout his career in West Michigan. He still lives in West Michigan with his wife. The couple has raised their two children and now enjoys their five grandchildren in the locations where they live. When not involved with his medical career, Dr. Harriman spends time with family and friends and enjoys running, reading, writing, sports, and being outdoors.